Hold My Beer and Watch This

Real Stories from a Small-Town ER

Volume 11

Kerry Hamm

Welcome to the emergency room! My name is Kerry, and for longer than I care to claim, I worked passionately and endlessly as an ER registration clerk. I have worked in both inner-city and small-town emergency rooms. To be honest, most of the chief complaints that presented at the larger hospital (in Virginia) were your typical complaints: car accidents, gunshot wounds, stab wounds, medical/jail clearances, and eight billion other patients looking for relief from colds or flus. The small-town hospital (in rural Ohio) is where most of the stories from my other books took place, and I can confidently tell you that the small town is where all the craziness was hiding all along. That was a primary reason to highlight stories from a small-town ER, as opposed to the inner city.

If you haven't read my previous books, don't worry; none of these books must be read in a specific order, as the stories included in each have occurred over a span of years.

This will be my final book in the '*Small-Town ER*' series, though I have every intention of continuing to sift through reader submissions and release books of others' encounters. One day, I may fully transition away from this genre, but for now, I enjoy reading submissions from readers, and I also enjoy interacting with my readers, most of whom are still in the medical field or have since retired, but want to relive that rush, even if for a moment. Most of these recollections didn't get passed to my previous books because they took place in an inner-city hospital. Some of these stories were long forgotten, popping up out of the blue when I met someone who reminded me of a previous patient or if I saw something on television that made me reflect on the past. A few, I must admit, simply did not make the cut for my other works because I didn't care much for them.

When I released the first book in this series, I didn't think I'd write a second. Now here we are, with more than ten volumes filled with stories of the past. I think it's about time that my own stories are put to rest, but someone out there will go to work every day, thinking 'That's the weirdest thing ever,' and go back the next thing to be proven wrong. Their stories will continue. The insanity will never end. Thank heavens for our EMTS, techs, doctors, police officers, firefighters, nurses, and anyone in the healthcare industry. These people keep our world turning.

In this book, I will leave most of the layout of the hospitals to your imagination, though you may refer to previous editions to read a loosely-based description of the rural hospital. Every story here is true, though dialogue has been changed slightly, all names have been changed, and some situations have been slightly altered to protect patient privacy. It has never been my intention to exploit the heartaches or embarrassments of others, but simply offer a glimpse into the world of the emergency room, where every patient is a wild card.

<u>Cheat Sheet</u>

Readers have brought to my attention that some of the terms I use in my books are confusing, meaning my readers can't fully enjoy the stories.

MVA: Motor Vehicle Accident

ETOH: ethyl alcohol is the real meaning of this, but in our ER this means our patient is drunk

CC/cc: chief complaint

Tones dropping: a series of melodic beeps play before dispatch alerts medics of a patient's call. Most of us groan when we hear the tones because we know we're getting another patient.

Stemi: a procedure in which a patient is taken to the Cath Lab to clear a cardiac blockage. From what I understand, this is done by making an incision near the groin rather than entering through the heart itself.

Face sheet/facesheet: a piece of paper detailing the patient's name, contact information, next of kin, primary physician, chief complaint, and insurance information. One copy must go to the back, the other to our tray. Then, another must go to medics, the floor (if a patient is admitted), and the coroner (if it comes down to that).

NOK: next of kin

DID: died in department

DOA: dead on arrival

BAC: blood alcohol content

Bus: another term for ambulance

LOC: level or consciousness or loss of consciousness, depending on context

If I have forgotten to include any terms you feel others may not recognize, feel free to leave a review with your suggestion!

The Illusive Leprechaun

I decided against telling this story in my previous books because I thought it sounded too harsh, and it happened at a not-so-small hospital. I've since decided against keeping it to myself, probably because I bumped into a woman who reminded me a lot of the patient involved in this story.

Mrs. X was a kind old woman. She always carried a plastic bag with candies her children purchased by the pound from a local grocery store. In all the times I'd seen her in the ER, I never saw her bag filled more than halfway. Mrs. X handed out wrapped caramels, butterscotch discs, and cinnamon balls like there was no tomorrow. It brought her joy, and none of the staff ever refused her tokens of appreciation.

We were all familiar with Mrs. X. She lived in an assisted living facility because she had dementia and was often confused. Her daughter once came to visit her in the ER and told us all that the decision to place Mrs. X in the facility was based upon Mrs. X setting her kitchen on fire when she attempted to microwave soup—while it was still in the can. Mrs. X could be introduced to a staff member 800 times, yet she wouldn't remember that person, even if only five minutes had passed between the staff member visiting her. This meant that Mrs. X's nurses, techs, and doctors usually ended up with pockets filled to the brims with candies by the time Mrs. X was either transferred to another wing or discharged back to her assisted living home.

During one particular visit to our ER, Mrs. X began handing out candy as usual. I was helping out the back by cleaning rooms and being a gopher, basically, so not only had I entered Mrs. X's room for registration purposes, but I also entered her room a few times to give her water, warm blankets, and pillows at her request. In that time, she'd insisted upon handing me candy after candy.

About an hour after Mrs. X arrived from her assisted living home, she exhibited behavior none of us had ever witnessed from her. She became bitter and noncompliant with staff members. She repeatedly pulled out her IV and kept unplugging machinery in her room. She even threw a pillow at one of the doctors. When she bit the x-ray tech, none of us knew how to react.

The charge nurse pulled me aside as I was running back and forth, and he asked me to call Mrs. X's daughter. It was three in the morning, and I felt horrible for having to make a phone call in the middle of the night, especially when phone calls from the hospital typically cause family members to panic, but the charge nurse believed Mrs. X's daughter could calm her enough for ER staff to finish labs and treatment.

Mrs. X's daughter was groggy when she answered the phone, but she was calm and polite.

"Oh gosh," she said, following my report of what was going down in the back. "I'll be there as soon as I can."

By the time Mrs. X's daughter made it across town, our patient was reacting so violently that the doctor ordered her to be restrained and security was dispatched to her room. She had taken to screaming about seeing a leprechaun in her room, and she threw a fit whenever staff came near her room, convinced the hospital staff members were teaming up with the leprechaun to terrorize her. She broke free from the staff attempting to restrain her and spit at anyone who moved too close. The decision was made to wait for her daughter to arrive.

Mrs. X's daughter entered the room and attempted to calm her mother, to no avail. Mrs. X did not seem to recognize her daughter. She shrieked and cried as she stood weakly and hunched over in the corner of the small room. The doctors on shift met for a pow-wow in the center of the nurses' station and decided that the best course of action would be to hold the patient down and administer a sedative. She would then most likely be admitted to mental health due to her condition and the security/safety measures the floor had to offer. It was quite a sad moment for all of us, who'd grown rather fond of Mrs. X and her generosity.

The patient fought tooth and nail when staff entered her room again. Her daughter was so upset by her mother's condition that she began sobbing and had to step outside to gather composure.

"He's after my gold!" Mrs. X shouted. She clutched her purse to her chest. "He keeps taking my jewelry!"

"Who?" asked one of the doctors.

"The leprechaun," she shouted. "He took my necklace and earrings, the ones with the pearls. He's after my gold! He took my candy, too, but you tell him that I'm reasonable. He can have it if he returns my gold."

As I went from room to room, gathering information from other patients, every last one of them showed concern for Mrs. X. None of them complained that they were left waiting, which I found to be a major relief in addition to it being a complete surprise that this group of patients understood the sadness and severity of the elderly Mrs. X's behavior.

Mrs. X was held down and given meds to ease her anxiety. She fought sleep and continued to mumble about the "mean little leprechaun" who'd been after her gold.

It wasn't too long after Mrs. X received her meds that we saw the 'leprechaun' to which our patient was referring.

"Hey," one of the doctors called to the lab tech headed toward Mrs. X's room, "have you been the one coming over to draw that patient's labs?"

The tech nodded. "Why?"

I stood next to the charge nurse, waiting for him to sign the paperwork I was supposed to fax to another hospital. I gently poked the charge nurse in the arm and nodded to the conversation the doctor was having with the lab tech.

Now would probably be a good idea to explain what the rest of us were seeing.

This lab tech, wearing lab's designated *green* scrubs, was a little person. He was new to our hospital, and night shift had only seen him a handful of times because he primarily worked day shift. None of us had been able to piece together Mrs. X's claims because the lab tech never came to mind.

Mrs. X's heart monitor's alert beeped rapidly when she set eyes on the lab tech. Though she had enough medication to keep her in bed, she still mustered the strength to shout out a few choice words, and she called for help.

"He's going to steal my gold!" she shouted in a raspy croak. She attempted to get out of bed, obviously headed to snatch her purse up, but she didn't have the energy to do so.

After security questioned the lab tech, the man admitted that he had gone through Mrs. X's purse and stolen some of her jewelry each time he had entered her room. It was discovered that he had been breaking up his visits to her room to cut down on the time she'd have to yell for help, so the labs he could have drawn in one visit to her room had been spaced out over a period of time to allow him to enter several times and steal one piece of jewelry each time. During his last visit to her room, he decided to take her candy and he'd stashed Mrs. X's wedding band in his blouse pocket.

The lab tech was terminated immediately following his confession and security notified the police department. As it would turn out, a few patients had filed complaints over the span of the lab tech's employment with our hospital, citing missing valuables. Once the house supervisor looked over the complaints, it was discovered that the lab tech had been linked to each of those patients' rooms. The lab tech was subsequently arrested on charges of theft. We heard he eventually admitted to other thefts and took a plea deal that would allow him to continue working in the field—just not at our hospital.

Following that night's drama, the ER staff pooled together to purchase Mrs. X a nice bouquet of flowers. Luckily, neither Mrs. X nor her daughter held a grudge against the ER staff.

Heard over the scanner during a full moon:

"We need an officer to respond to a call from two subjects on Alphabet Road. They claim they are being held hostage in their vehicle by an angry goose. Transport required for one passenger. She said she got out of the car and tried to shoo it away, but it bit her."

What Time Do You Have?

A man, probably in his early or mid-twenties, once arrived at the ER registration desk at four in the morning. He was told to arrive at five for a procedure, so I explained to the man that he was early and that the surgical department staff had not yet arrived. Boy, was this man irate. Though a security guard was sitting next to me, the man was undeterred from exhibiting callous behavior. He called me every name in the book, and when security tried to calm the man, he called the guard every name in the second book of the series, *'Every Insult Known to Man.'*

The patient demanded that I register him and send him to the surgical unit, but I couldn't. Our system was set up in a way that the man was pre-registered, but I couldn't do anything with his account until it was actually time for the surgery to take place. Our system was set up that way to make the hospital more accountable for time and billing, so my hands were tied. In addition to this, I could not send the man to that wing of the hospital because we were not allowed to leave patients in unattended areas in instances like this one.

"I just drove here from Kentucky," he declared. "I left at four. It took an hour to get here. Register me and get me over there now."

I kind of looked at the man. "Sir, your residence is located in a different time zone than the hospital."

"But I drove an hour to get here. My watch says it's now after five. I'm going to be late because you can't do your job right."

I shook my head and tried to explain that because of the time zones, though the man did drive for an hour, it still wasn't 5:00 where he was now.

"That makes no sense!" he shouted. His face was turning red and I thought he was going to have an anger-induced stroke right there in front of me.

The security guard attempted to explain the time zone to the gentleman, but he still wasn't grasping the concept. In his mind, he was right and we were not only wrong, but also stupid for coming up with some asinine excuse as to why we couldn't help him at that time.

A nurse in the back heard the commotion and came to the front to check it out. She apparently knew the guy's mother and threatened to call his mother if he wouldn't sit in the waiting room and wait until it was time to register.

The nursing supervisor received a complaint a few days following the man's surgery, and she wanted to know why I kept the man waiting for an hour over his scheduled procedure time. Once I explained the situation, she laughed and told me not to worry.

<u>Repetition</u>

Some people, I think, live their lives in repetition. Come to think of it, most of us do, right? I wake up around the same time each day, walk and feed the animals, work or goof around, stay up way too late, and then get up and do it all over again. Most of us follow a routine for our daily lives. I'd go as far to say that sometimes we feel like we have mundane routines, but when you take a moment to imagine the repetition others follow, you'll see your daily routine isn't so bad after all.

Mr. Smith was back for pain meds for the fifth time that week, and he hadn't become any more pleasant than he was when I registered him the day before. He swore his roommate stole his pills. Last time, the bottle of Percocet was stolen by his landlord, so Mr. Smith didn't appear to have trustworthy acquaintances.

The anxiousness Mr. Smith was presenting with was not atypical behavior. He admitted he used (and abused) recreational drugs. He would often present with injuries that the staff believed he caused to himself, hoping to score another prescription. Just a week earlier, he came in with a nearly-severed finger. He said he slammed his finger in the door of a car. What he wouldn't say is if he did that on purpose or accident. A lot of us thought it was the previous, based on the man's behavior in the year he'd been a frequent flyer.

That night, the ER was packed. The weather wasn't particularly great. It wasn't the worst we'd ever seen near the coast, but MVAs were coming in by the handfuls every few minutes, and the charge nurse had to call in reinforcements.

Mr. Smith paced the lobby and picked at his skin. He checked the wall clock every six minutes—on the dot. He nervously glanced out the windows every few minutes. When he heard our police scanner sound off, he actually leaned in to hear what dispatch and the officers were saying. The four clerks at the desk couldn't even pay attention to the scanner because it was so busy.

The operator called and transferred a call from the cops to my line.

"You wouldn't have seen Mr. Smith tonight, would you?"

"Yes," I responded. "Right here, right now."

"Don't agitate him tonight," the officer instructed. "Try to move him someplace where he won't see us coming."

"Will do," I said.

I pretended to take paperwork to the security office and let the two guards inside know that the cops were headed our direction. Mr. Smith had a routine set aside in his life for police involvement as well, and it was a strict routine that I like to call 'See the cops and run.'

Security notified the charge nurse of all of this and I was instructed to take Mr. Smith down to the cafeteria. He always demanded a sandwich following his treatment or denial of pain meds, so I was told to just tell him we were treating him to the sandwich first due to how busy we were. It made sense at the time.

Everything was fine at first. Mr. Smith first seemed irritated that he would have to wait longer to tell his sob story, but he was thrilled that he was getting VIP treatment and escorted to the now-closed-to-public cafeteria.

His cooperation was short-lived.

The cops never told me how close they were to the hospital, and we didn't get Mr. Smith moved to an isolated location quick enough. As soon as he saw the flashing lights reflecting off our white walls, he took off down the crowded hall, dodging foot traffic and even knocking down an orderly.

One of the security guards groaned as he ran by the registration desk.

The cops weren't playing around that night, and I couldn't blame them for not wanting to.

We knew things were about to get *real fun* the moment we saw those front paws lean out of the patrol car and hit the parking lot pavement. The K-9 officer was itching to catch herself a bad guy.

Three officers and two security guards chased the man down the halls. He thought he could elude the officers by hopping in an elevator, but the thing about this was pretty simple: the arrows above the elevators showed what floor the man was on. He rode up to the ninth floor, then the tenth, and then rode back down again to the first floor. We could all hear the K-9 handler warn that he was going to release the dog if the man tried to run, and I guess Mr. Smith saw that as a challenge. It was only his third run-in with the dog that year, and I suppose he was determined to win at least one round against the four-legged officer.

Unsurprisingly, Mr. Smith didn't win this round with the dog, either. Patients and family members from the waiting room gathered in the halls to watch the K-9 clamp down on Mr. Smith's forearm, and when the man began screaming, some of the bystanders laughed, while others cringed.

The cops revealed that Mr. Smith tried to sell his pills to an undercover officer. He escaped arrest and headed to our hospital in an attempt to procure more meds.

I don't exactly know how the law continued to fail the innocent and protect the guilty, but Mr. Smith served something like two or three days of jail time before he was released. He was expected to show up for multiple court days that stemmed from all his run-ins with the cops, but he saw the officers early when he tried to rob a gas station. Only then was he locked up for a long while.

I tell you what, I'd rather have my boring routine over getting bitten by a K-9 unit any day.

Shark Bait (Ooh-ha-Never Mind)

A rather intoxicated man registered just before midnight with a shark bite to his hand. The shark had gotten the man good, too. A chunk of flesh was missing out of the side of his left palm, and the skin surrounding the bite appeared fileted. My coworker placed the patient on our board and called to the back to notify someone of the profusely-bleeding bite.

Our head nurse called up and I answered.

"Kerry, do me a favor and find out what bay he was in. I'm so busy back here that I've been holding my pee for, like, three hours. When he tells you, go ahead and call the wildlife number. I'll have Wanda run that up to you when I can find her."

"Will do," I said.

I looked to the man who was sitting in a wheelchair next to the ER entrance. "Sir, what bay were you in when this happened?"

"Huh?"

"We report injuries like this to a wildlife department. They keep track of them for, like, statistics or something. So, were you out by Alphabet Bay when this happened?"

He was still confused. "Uh…no?"

"Oh," I answered. "I just figured you were because it's the closest. Do you remember what bay you were in?"

He blinked at me like I was stupid. "I wasn't in a bay. I was in my bathroom."

"You sustained a shark bite while you were in your bathroom?" I asked. I started the think the man was too drunk to respond properly. After all, he reeked of vodka and was dropped off by a taxi.

He nodded. "Yeah. I keep it in my bathtub."

It took a second for me to realize the man was serious, but my words still came out in a wild exclamation. "You keep a shark in your bathtub?"

Yes. Yes, the man somehow became the proud owner of a bull shark calf and was keeping it in his bathtub. He told the police that he didn't know what he was going to do with it when it outgrew the tub, but for the time being, he had been feeding it live fish and raw hamburger.

Since that moment, I've met people who've owned gigantic snakes (like the one that escaped in our hospital that one time), kept alligators in their tubs, and even someone who owned a lion. I'll never really understand that, but I've still been shocked each and every time these people have told me what animals they kept as pets.

<u>My Business</u>

Someone once told me that I had no reason to listen to the police scanner because the events were "none of my business." I know for a fact that one night the scanner helped me out because the neighbors had called in a disturbance occurring at my residence. My neighbors could not remember where I worked, so when I heard dispatch announce my address and possible home intruders as I was sitting across town at the ER registration desk, I was able to call the police and find out information. True story, hand to God. Luckily, I was informed that my dogs seemed to have scared off the possible intruders. I thanked my neighbors for their vigilance in our neighborhood watch program.

Indeed, the scanner feed aided registration, security, and the nurses many times. I do believe I detailed in a previous book how registration heard over the scanner about a problematic group of family members, all of whom arrived in an uproar. Nobody had alerted our security guards, so we were able to do so and have the guards at our sides. The police did not arrive to the hospital for some time later due to whatever they were doing, so having the scanner feed allowed us to page security and secure the registration area, which was, indeed, much needed.

Not long after I left the small-town hospital loosely depicted in my previous books, something scary happened. I had been listening to the scanner off and on throughout the night, mostly out of habit. Not too much had been going on around town. The police department still had a BOLO (be on the lookout) for a subject, but nobody said the subject's name or why the subject was wanted. At one point, I turned the feed off in order to watch a movie.

Midway through the movie, which was a horror, by the way, someone walked by my living room window and peered inside. I'm not sure where horror film directors got the idea that main characters shriek like little girls during scary moments, because when I'm scared—like I was then—I tend to jump and blurt out just about every single curse word I know in one big run-on jumble. There's no screaming involved, but rest assured that if there are kids around when I'm scared, they're going to learn some new words. I called for the dogs and rushed to the front and back doors to make sure they were locked.

As I was running around the house like a chicken with my head cut off, searching for my cordless phone, I heard voices on my front porch and thought I heard a man talking at the back of my house. Of course, my dogs were barking nonstop, and I could hardly hear a man repeat three times that he was with the police department. I peeked out the window and saw officers shining spotlights between houses on the block and in an open field across the street. I could see lights shining in my backyard, and two officers were on my front porch, waiting for me to open the door.

"Hey," said one officer, as the other stepped off the porch to do a perimeter check of my residence, "has anyone been by your house recently?"

I nodded. My heart was practically barely hanging on, about to jump right out of my chest. I had goosebumps running up and down my arms. The dogs were still barking, and my mind was racing.

The officer glanced over my head and into what little he could see of the kitchen. He asked in a whisper, "Has anyone entered your home within the last few minutes?"

I shook my head. "No, but someone just walked by and looked in my window," I answered, motioning to the front of the house.

"Did you hear your car doors open or close, or did you hear your doorknobs or windows rattling, like someone was trying to get in?"

I thought for a second. "Not that I recall. I was watching a scary movie and—."

"You're watching a scary movie at two in the morning?" the officer asked.

"Well, yeah," I said with a light laugh.

"Okay," he said. "Sorry to cut you off. What happened?"

I explained, "Well, it was right at the part in the movie where you just know something's about to jump out and scare you, so I was already on edge about that, but some guy just walked right by the window and looked inside. And I mean, he was in the yard. He wasn't walking on the sidewalk."

"Get a good look at him?"

I shook my head. "Not really. It scared me so much just to see someone there that I kind of flipped out, and when he saw that I saw him, he kind of took off pretty quickly."

The officer sighed. "We're going to have some officers patrolling down here for a while, but you should probably stay inside for the night."

"Uh, okay…"

The officer thanked me for my time and reminded me to lock the door once I closed it.

Not once did anyone tell me who they were looking for or why. I recognized the officer I spoke with from my time at the hospital, though he and I only rarely saw one another back then. I still think I would have gotten more information if the other officer(s) had been the one(s) to speak with me, just because they knew my history.

Thankfully, one of the security guards from the hospital contacted me and asked if I was okay. I said I was, but the cops had just left and would be patrolling my area throughout the rest of the night.

"Did they tell you who they were looking for?"

"Nope."

"Your buddy."

"Which one?" I laughed. At first, I thought the guard was making a joke and would just say the name of one of the frequent flyers who'd also been in trouble with law enforcement.

"Remember that guy who left those Christmas presents at your house?"

I froze. "I thought he was still in jail."

"Not as far as I know. I guess he just got out like yesterday or today."

"They think it's him?"

"They said his name. He was here earlier. Asked about you, too. We didn't tell him anything."

"Why were the cops looking for him?"

"He busted out someone's car window, like, a block from your house and then the cops saw him go down your street. They lost him, though."

Thankfully, someone was kind enough to tell me what was going on. I did not go outside that night, and I probably don't have to tell any of you that I also did not sleep that night.

I found out the man in question was picked up just about half a block from my house. He was found hiding on someone's front porch.

I, for one, fully support our local scanner feeds. You just never know when they'll be able to help you out.

Citizen's Arrest...Arrest

I remember being called in early one night and four squad cars were parked in front of the ER entrance. Since we were in the city, I didn't give it much thought. I figured they were responding to a violent patient or something of the sort.

When I walked inside, I passed several patients in our out-in-the-open waiting room. Many of them had surely been hit with the winter bug that was going around, as they were all hacking up their lungs. One woman held an ice pack to a bruise on her face. A man held a wailing baby.

At the registration window, four officers stood in a single-file line, each accompanying a male in handcuffs.

"Didn't your shift just start?" I asked one of the officers.

"It's gonna be a long night," he said, with a roll of his eyes. "Geniuses here decided to rob a store."

"Wow. All four?"

"Hey," the last guy in line said. "Don't you group me in with them. I didn't rob nobody. I was making a citizen's arrest."

"My bad," the cop corrected. "That one," he pointed, "witnessed the robbery, so he pulled out his own gun and went chasing after these other three."

"So why is he under arrest? It's not illegal to help, right?"

"Exactly!" the guy at the end yelled. "I was doing what any good citizen would do. You wouldn't even know where these three ran off to unless I went chasing after them."

"Yeah," said one of the other criminals at the middle of the line. "And you can bet that once we're all booked that we're going to thank you for that."

"Are you making threats while you're in custody?" another officer asked his prisoner.

The man shook his head. "Nope. Just making promises."

"You guys are going to put my life on the line, when all I was doing was the right thing?" the man at the back asked.

I groaned. So much drama was happening within my first three minutes in the building, and it was a fair indication that the ER was going to be hopping.

"Why don't you just explain what you were arrested for, before you decided to try to run from us?"

The man mumbled something incoherent.

"This one," the officer explained, "did try to do the right thing. It just turns out that he had three outstanding warrants for his own attempted robbery."

"So…a robber trying to stop other robbers?"

"Hey," the guy said with a snarl. "You know what? I was robbing the DMV. These dudes were robbing a grocery store. You can't tell me that the DMV doesn't deserve to get robbed. But these guys, they were screaming and pointing guns at pregnant women and yelling at kids and stuff."

I nodded. "So valiant of you to take a stand."

"We rolled up and recognized our guy here, so when we told him he was under arrest—."

"He ran?"

The officer nodded. "He did."

The man sighed. "Only reason I got caught was because I slipped on some ice."

"And when he slipped he shot the window out of another business. So, we have him on his warrants, felony firearm possession, and destroying property."

"And running from the cops," the guy added.

Most embarrassing shift EV-ER:

I'd worked for two hours before someone stopped me in the hall and told me I had something static-clung to my sweater.

People, it was a thong.

My coworkers let me walk around for TWO HOURS with a THONG stuck to my back.

D.U.H. Er, D.U.I

On a rather slow overnight shift, our security guards, some of the nurses and techs from the back, and I were up front, listening to the scanner feed. Officers had been in a high-speed pursuit with a subject responsible for slamming into a parked car. They'd somehow lost the subject on a dirt road.

We all turned the scanner off, thinking the hype was over, and we took to browsing the internet or watching movies on one of the guards' tablets. In the back, the nurses were listening to loud music with the lights dimmed. Someone went upstairs and stole doughnuts from ICU's break room. It was one big party down in the ER.

That soon ended when two officers literally dragged a kicking, spitting, and screaming woman through the ER doors.

"Call back there and tell someone to get me a stretcher," one of the officers ordered me.

The security guard at my side jumped right up, leaving *The Longest Yard* playing in the background. He stat-paged his partner as I called to the back.

"Thank you for calling Road Kill Express. You kill it, we grill it."

I chuckled. "Hey. We need a bed up front. Cops are here."

The female was screaming at the top of her lungs.

"Gee, what's wrong with that one?"

"Pretty sure she's resisting," I answered.

"And we deployed pepper spray."

"And the cop said—."

She groaned. "Oh, for Pete's sake. I heard him. We'll be up in a minute."

The woman tried to roll around on the floor as the officers each held one of her arms.

"I'm going to put you down for a minute," one officer said. "You're going to stay right there until these nice ladies get you on a stretcher and all cleaned up."

Both officers released the subject.

Want to know what she *didn't* do? She didn't 'stay right there.'

No sooner than the officers released the woman did she hop up and try to run out the ER doors. Because the doors were not set up like typical sliding doors, but only opened on one side, the woman ran smack-dab into the glass. While she was sobbing and kicking the door in frustration, the officers were laughing so hard they were almost crying, too.

"It's not funny!" she shouted, only using a string of expletives in that statement. "These jerks maced me. I didn't do crap wrong!"

That's when one officer went from laughing to taking a deep, angry sigh. "You didn't do anything wrong? Jane, do you know how many lives you put in danger by making us chase you through town tonight?"

"I don't care," she yelled.

"Well, that's apparent."

"I didn't do anything wrong," the woman repeated.

"You know how we caught her?" the other officer asked me, still chuckling.

I shook my head. "We turned off the scanner when you lost her."

"This dimwit tried to back up into someone's driveway."

I wasn't following. "And that's how you caught her?"

"No!" the officer blurted out, doubling over as tears streamed down his cheeks.

"Don't you dare tell anyone," the woman yelled.

The officer started to speak again, when the woman charged at him, because *that's* always a good idea. He knocked her to the ground with one arm just as two nurses wheeled a bed to the lobby.

"She backed her car up through someone's house," the other officer explained, as the one who'd knocked the subject down checked on her.

"Oh my," I responded. "Like, through the house?"

He nodded. "They woke up and found a car in their front room."

"Holy crap."

The woman continued to fight as the nurses, officers, and security attempted to place her on the bed. After nearly 10 minutes of the woman resisting, the charge nurse came up front and used her 'boss' voice. The woman cried and protested momentarily, but then willingly climbed on the bed.

Lab results came back for the woman. Not only was her BAC twice the legal limit, but she also confessed to using bath salts. It wasn't shocking in the least to hear that the woman did not have car insurance. She did have an outstanding warrant in the next county over, though.

Police officers brought in a completely-naked woman at two in the morning. She was a medical clearance following being tackled and complaining of arm pain. She told me she had been running through the cemetery nude because she was born naked and would die naked.

She tested positive for LSD and her BAC was .4-something.

The Sting

The nursing supervisor unexpectedly showed up at the registration desk, accompanied by our security guards. My coworker and I hadn't been doing much that night, unless you count creating boards on Pinterest as doing a lot.

"We're about to get some patients in here, and there are going to be lots of officers. You're probably going to see firefighters, too."

"Uh, okay," I stated.

"You're going to let everyone in and out as they need to come and go," she continued.

I nodded, confused because it was common practice in the ER to allow law enforcement and first responders to do as they please. As you're all aware, having emergency responders in the ER is not abnormal in the slightest, so I wasn't quite sure why the nursing supervisor was telling us this.

"Now, security is going to stay with you, and some of the officers said they're going to be in the area. Some will be in plain clothes. They said they will have uniformed officers in the triage area."

"Okay," I said. "What's going on right now?"

"Nothing good," the supervisor responded.

"Meaning?" asked my coworker.

"Meaning a pair of criminals were involved in breaking and entering, and the cops are trying to catch the rest of their group."

I was still confused, but the supervisor didn't have time to explain further. She hightailed it to the back just as two ambulances pulled in the lot. Each ambulance had its lights and sirens going, a sure sign that what the RNs were about to see wasn't going to be a pretty sight.

Two males presented to the ER with multiple gunshot wounds to their abdomens and legs. My coworker and I worked with the unit clerk to get the patients in the system, and we also worked to contact the transferring helicopter service.

Just like the nursing supervisor said, a slew of officers and firefighters arrived to the ER. We popped the doors and allowed each of them to visit the patients' rooms. And, like the supervisor said, more officers came in and informed us they were going to be in the triage room. Plain clothes officers arrived and walked straight to the waiting room, where they sat and appeared to be your average family member, impatiently waiting for a patient to be discharged from the back.

We still had no idea what was happening, and it was rather unsettling. This part of Ohio doesn't see gang activity. Gunshot wounds are few and far between. To my knowledge, this was the first 'sting' the hospital had ever seen.

"Did they tell you guys anything?" I whispered to one of the security guards.

"Just that the guys in the back were trying to rob a house. Something went wrong, they were loaded up with bullets, and now the cops are trying to get the other people involved to come in."

"How do they know there are other people involved?"

"Guess the guys in back ratted on them. The cops said they could probably work out a deal if they could get the others to come in, so they let the guys call their buddies, and now we're just waiting. We're supposed to act like we don't know what's going on, though."

I bit my lip. "Are these people going to cause trouble?"

The guard shrugged. "Dunno. Cops think so, but dunno. Don't worry, though. You two just stay calm. We're right here, and you have officers surrounding you. They're trained for stuff like this."

As we waited, we gathered that the patients' buddies were not so much considered a 'gang,' but they were involved in a string of violent robberies that extended across the state. Two of the friends owned a business that required traveling, and the group of friends got the bright idea to commit crimes while out of our area, believing they were less likely to get caught. They were right. Their line of crimes in other counties remained unsolved. This boosted their egos, and the men went from petty crimes of stealing from homes while residents were gone shopping to breaking in occupied residences and businesses, holding families and patrons at gunpoint.

From what I understood, the men in the back simply chose the wrong house to enter in the middle of the night. The owner shot both men, and in the confusion and panic of the situation, the men somehow ended up shooting each other. Realizing they were in some deep doo-doo, the men agreed to rat out their friends. They called their buddies up and apparently told them they were involved in a car wreck, so the rest of the criminals had no idea the men had really been shot and were now under arrest.

To be quite honest, the rest of this story was fairly uneventful. A group of three men arrived to the ER lobby and inquired about the patients. We confirmed their identities and officers swooped in and arrested the men. Two of the men were carrying firearms but never attempted to use them. One man voluntarily dropped to the ground and told his arresting officer that he knew it was only a matter of time before the group was caught. The whole thing lasted like two minutes, if that.

As far as I'm aware, all the men involved were sentenced to lengthy prison sentences.

Heard over the scanner at three in the morning:

"We need a few officers to respond to Burger King. I've received reports of a group of teenagers licking the outside windows."

Hang in There

One of the strangest things I've ever witnessed happened when I was leaving an unplanned double shift. As I was walking out, a woman sped through our parking lot, threw her car in park at the ER entrance, and bolted from the still-running vehicle. She shouted for help.

None of that sounds out of the ordinary, right?

Well, hanging out of her passenger window was a rail-thin man. He was kicking his feet in the air. His upper body was inside the car, while his pelvis and legs hanged outside the vehicle.

I had just worked sixteen hours. You can bet I sure wasn't getting involved in that crap-show.

Bystanders rushed to the vehicle and security came outside.

"What's this?" one of the guards asked the driver.

"I had my windows rolled down and he tried to climb inside my car when I was stopped at a light," the woman frantically explained.

She didn't know what else to do in that moment, except for rolling up the window in a desperate attempt to keep him out of the car. Rather than pull away, the man continued to crawl inside. Realizing the man wasn't going to give up, the woman rolled the passenger window up until the man was caught between the glass and the seal. She kept one finger on the window button and drove two blocks to the hospital—with the man hanging out of her car.

My coworkers told me the man was arrested without injuries, but he tested positive for meth. He couldn't tell anyone exactly why he tried to enter the woman's vehicle, though I'm sure it wasn't for the purpose of making a new friend. The 'passenger' went to jail and the driver was sent on her way.

So, I bumped into one of our local police officers the other day and asked him how he's been. He shook his head, sighed, and said, "I just responded to a call from a man who called 911 to report his girlfriend took all of his heroin and left. You can just guess how I've been."

<u>No Visitors</u>

A woman rushed inside, following an
ambulance pulling in our bay. The woman
was crying uncontrollably and we could
barely understand her. It took about five
minutes for her to calm down enough to tell
us why she was there.

"My boyfriend," she sobbed, "is hurt. I
hurt him."

We worked with the woman for another
few minutes to get her boyfriend's name and
confirmed he was the patient transported in
the latest ambulance.

"I need to see him. I need to tell him I'm
sorry. It was an accident."

She stopped crying in an instant and
jumped up from her seat in the lobby.

"Oh my God," she said. "I'm going to
get arrested. They're going to put me in jail
and I'll lose my job. And if I lose my job,
I'll be homeless. And I'll lose my car. I'll

have to live on the streets. It was an accident. You have to tell them it was an accident. Please. Please, go back there and tell everyone it was an accident. I can't go to jail over this. Please. Just let me see him so I can explain that I didn't do this on purpose."

"I'll go check on his condition and see if you can go back," I assured the woman.

"Hey," I said to the charge nurse, when I went to the back. "What's up with the new guy in the trauma room?"

"He got shot."

"Like, a gunshot?"

The charge nurse shook her head. "Nail gun."

"Really? Well, his girlfriend is freaking out in the lobby. She wants to know if she can come back."

"I don't really care," said the nurse. "Just check with the patient first."

I nodded and went to the man's room.

Sticking straight out of the center of his chest was a long, shiny silver nail. His shirt was saturated with blood, and the man was breathing rapidly, while exhaling in heavy huffs.

"Knock, knock," I said, lightly tapping on the room's open door.

"Are you going to take this out?"

I shook my head. "Just registration. Your girlfriend sent me back to—."

"That-that…She is *not* my girlfriend," the man growled. "That woman is absolutely psychotic. I don't want her near me."

I offered a nervous chuckle. "Well, that answers my question."

"I want to press charges," the man informed me. "Can you call the cops? I asked the lady on the ambulance, but she said to tell you guys."

I nodded. "I'll track down your nurse and tell her you would like the police to be notified. That's really no trouble at all."

"Do not let that crazy woman back here. She is certifiable. I don't even really know her, you know? She sent me a friend request on Facebook and we had mutual friends, so I thought maybe I knew her through them, but

I didn't. So, she started sending me all of these weird messages. Then, she started messaging my wife, telling my wife that I was having an affair. I swear to God, I don't even know this woman. I went to work today, and this lady just...she just showed up!"

"She knew where you worked?"

"I mean, I deleted her from Facebook after she messaged my wife, but I put on my page that I work for XYZ Construction, so, I mean, I guess? What I don't know is how she knew I was at that site. My wife didn't even know the address to that site. This psycho...You know, I think she's stalking me."

I told the man the woman in the lobby was sobbing and said she shot the man by accident, but that made him even more frustrated.

"That's a boldfaced lie," he blurted out. "I told her to leave, so she picked up my nail gun and aimed it right at me. She said she was tired of me disrespecting her, so she shot me. This thing isn't by my heart, is it?

Am I going to die? Can you call my wife? My wife doesn't know I'm here."

I agreed to calling the patient's wife. I also notified the patient's nurse of the man's story and was subsequently ordered to notify security. The patient's nurse told me to go back to the front and simply tell the woman that the patient was not stable enough for visitors, but if the man's wife showed up, escort her to the back. We both hoped the police would arrive before the patient's wife, just to avoid a conflict between the two.

Yeah, that didn't work.

When I called the patient's wife, she told me she was at a gas station located a block away, and she arrived within two minutes of us hanging up. Of course, she walked right up to the registration area and asked for her husband by name.

"You can just follow me," I said to her in a low voice.

The woman in the lobby stood. "But you told me he can't have visitors."

She pointed to the patient's wife. "And just who are you?"

I tried to rush the wife to the back, but she replied, "I'm John's wife. Who are— You're that crazy lady! What are you even *doing* here?"

"I'm Johnny's girlfriend. You have no right to be here."

"Ma'am," I said to the patient's wife. "Please follow me."

She shook her head. "No. I want this woman gone. Now."

"I'm not leaving," the other woman snapped. "He loves me and wants me here."

Right as the women approached each other, just as I thought there was going to be a massive brawl in the lobby, security stepped in and the police arrived.

The woman in the lobby was wanted for felony stalking and was arrested. The patient with the nail in his chest lived and did not require surgery. Someone in the back told me the nail had just pierced his chest and the blood was from a nicked vessel.

Eye Don't Want to Deal with You

My coworkers were about to clock out for the night. I had a feeling that as soon as they all left, crap was going to hit the fan and the ER was going to get slammed. That's usually how it worked. So, as soon as my coworkers punched out and exited the building, I can't say I was a bit surprised to see two adults entering the ER lobby with six children—probably ranging in age from two to eight—trailing behind them.

"How much do you want to be that they're all going to be seen?" the triage nurse joked under her breath.

"I'm not betting against you because you're probably right," I replied.

Mom stepped to the counter with one of two sons. Her hands were trembling and her voice was shaky. I glanced over at the boy's father and the child's siblings. Some had taken to crying, while the father was staring off at highlights of an earlier football game.

"We, uh, have a problem," said the mother.

"Let's start with a name and some identifying information," I said. "Then we'll get registered."

"I don't think we can wait for all that," the mom said, raising her voice. "Look, I thought this was the emergency room? Why do you make people wait if you're going to put up a huge sign saying to come here for emergencies?"

I wasn't quite sure what type of emergency we were looking forward to. The six-year-old wasn't crying. He wasn't doubled over in pain. He was capable of walking unassisted. Neither the triage nurse nor I could detect the presence of blood.

So, let's hear it. What type of emergency were we looking at, that the mother could waste time to demand to be seen immediately, when she could have used those few seconds to just give me the information I needed?

"What's the emergency?" asked the triage nurse. Her words came out dryer than she intended, but I couldn't blame her. She was on hour thirteen of an eighteen-hour shift.

"Maybe we should just go someplace else," said the mother, only her words sounded like a threatening question.

"Ma'am, we can help your son. We just need to know what type of emergency he's having."

"If she's going to sit around, asking for stupid information," the mother said, pointing at me, "and you're going to talk to me like that, I really don't know if I want my son seen here. Maybe we should just drive the forty minutes to the other hospital."

Those threats always left me befuddled. It was such an emergency that this mother couldn't be bothered to simply give me her son's name and date of birth, but she could drive forty minutes for him to be treated elsewhere.

"That's your choice," the triage nurse replied. "But if you would like to have your son treated here, just know that we'll need to have him registered before we can offer an examination or treatment. This young lady will just need his birth—."

"FINE," screamed the mother. Her other five children were racing each other down the empty corridor. I'm not sure where dad went, but he was out of sight. "He was born in 2007. December."

"And his name?"

"She just said you needed his birthday. See? I could be halfway to that other place by now."

The triage nurse and I both sighed at the same time.

"John Smith," the mother snapped. She began talking to herself. "I have never met anyone in the healthcare industry as rude and unprofessional as you two are. And you call yourselves an emergency room. Yeah, right."

"And John's birthday?"

"I already *told* you his birthday."

"Ma'am," I gently explained, "I have eleven patients named John Smith who were born in December of 2007. Our records are linked with area hospitals."

"So, pick the one in our town."

I blinked.

Even if I picked 'our' town, which was not guaranteed to be *her* town, I still had four results.

And, as I suspected, the mother finally screamed the name of a nearby town, not the one in which our hospital was located.

She became agitated once more when I asked what type of emergency her son was having, so I simply typed UNKNOWN in the chief complaint slot. We'd find out soon enough, anyway. She was cussing up a storm as the triage nurse escorted her and her son to the triage room.

"Honey, how'd you get that in there?" I heard the triage nurse ask.

"Does that even matter?" mom griped. "How 'bout you do your job and just take it out?"

The triage nurse did not take the patient straight back, but instead completed the triage process, that took about ten minutes longer than it usually did because the child's mother wouldn't shut up and stop complaining. Finally, the child was taken to a non-trauma room.

Just a few minutes later, the patient's nurse called me and informed me that I needed to gather the patient's information, as a doctor from Peds was coming down, and I would likely not be interested in going in the room during that time.

The situation during this process was irritatingly similar to the scene up front. Halfway through asking normal questions, I gave up. The child's mother refused to cooperate, and nobody could find the child's father, even after a complaint was made to security that the patient's siblings were running wild and climbing on the waiting room furniture. I made a note on the account that the mother refused to either correct or verify existing information.

"Have fun," the patient's nurse whispered to the Peds doc as I was leaving the room and he was going in.

He took a deep, cleansing breath to prepare himself.

"Did you see it?" the patient's nurse asked me.

I shook my head. "What was it?"

"He stuck one of his sister's press-on earrings to his eyeball because he wanted to have contacts like some kid at his school."

"Wouldn't that just fall out of his eye?"

"I would have thought so," the nurse responded. "Didn't, though. It's suctioned right on there."

The Peds doctor was able to remove the hard and thick, jewel-shaped sticker from the child's eye after administering half a bottle of eye drops and massaging the child's eye. The boy sustained heavy scratching to his cornea and left the ER with an eye patch.

Now, I know you probably couldn't believe it after mom's fantastic behavior during the visit, but she was just as angry leaving as she was while she was there. This time, she was complaining that she shouldn't get a bill for something she could have easily done at home.

Sticky Situation

A mother brought in her toddler one afternoon. Yes, the child was crying and wildly extending her hand, but the girl's mother was the one truly freaking out. She was bawling so hard she gagged and eventually vomited on the new rug housekeeping had placed at the registration window only an hour earlier. I couldn't understand a single thing she was saying to me, and nothing I said would calm her down. If you were there, you'd probably think that the mother had just been handed a death sentence.

A triage nurse directed the patient's mother to sit in a wheelchair and took the two back to a room, passing over the traditional triage process. Mom was given a few Valium, and the child's hand was placed in a bowl of acetone to remove the super glue that had bonded her fingers together.

That's it. That was what mom was panicking about.

"I swear, I just ran to the bathroom. When I came out, she had glue all over the floor and her fingers!" the mom said. She was still crying when she left the ER, but her daughter was happy again and must have waved goodbye to the nurses, registration staff, patients in the waiting room, and security guards about five thousand times in twenty seconds.

Piece it Together

I pointed to the sidewalk outside of the ER doors and asked security, "What's that guy doing?"

The guard shrugged. "He looks drunk."

"Should I go out there with a wheelchair?"

"Just let him come in first. You don't know if he's aggressive or not."

"So, shouldn't you check?"

"Eh, just let him come inside."

The man was staggering. He'd take two steps forward and one giant near-fall back.

Our triage nurse arrived to the registration desk. She took a bite of her cookie and nodded upward. "What's up with him?"

"I think he's drunk," the guard responded.

"What's that thing on his arm?"

I leaned over to better inspect the security cameras.

"Don't know. It's white, though."

"I see that," the nurse nodded.

"I should take a wheelchair out," I repeated.

"No," the nurse rushed. "You don't know if he's violent. Let me finish my cookie, and I'll go out there."

"Fine," the security guard huffed, "I'll go."

The triage nurse shrugged and continued with her cookie, while the security guard wheeled a chair outside and directed the man to sit. We could tell it wasn't going so well out there. The man was waving his arms and kept grabbing the brick exterior for support, all while yelling words we couldn't quite make out over the sound of the doors opening and closing repeatedly.

"Yeah, he's gotta be drunk," said the triage nurse. "Call back and tell them to get one of the orderlies up here for an ETOH."

I did as I was instructed and the orderly came to the front.

"Where are they?" he asked.

The triage nurse and I silently pointed to the entrance. Our security guard was still arguing with the man about sitting in the wheelchair.

After a few minutes of the orderly joining in, both hospital employees gave up and instead closely followed the man inside. The security guard's face was red from holding in laughter, while the orderly just let giggles fly.

"What's that on his arm?" asked the triage nurse, as the man staggered nearer to us.

"Let him show you," our guard replied with a snicker.

"Come on up here, sir. What brings you in tonight?"

The man, probably in his mid-thirties, stopped walking, but still swayed. He turned his head and pointed. "A car."

I chuckled.

"No," said the triage nurse. "Why did you come here tonight?"

The man belched and a poison cloud of alcohol drifted through the lobby and behind the ER desk. I gagged.

"This," the man said, pointing to his right arm.

"John," the nurse said to the orderly, "I left my glasses in the back. What is that thing?"

"It's a pipe!" the drunk man exclaimed.

Yes, it sure was a pipe. The man had a PVC pipe joint stuck around his forearm.

"Sir, why do you have a pipe on your arm?"

The man fell forward and smacked his head on the edge of the registration desk. I gasped. The nurse, security guard, and orderly basically picked the man up from the floor and shoved him in a wheelchair.

"It's stuck," the man said with a slur, paying no mind to the fact that he just almost knocked himself out.

"Why'd you put your arm through a pipe?"

"I don't know!" he shouted. "But I can't get it off!"

I had to call the fire department at four in the morning because our hospital didn't have the tools necessary to remove the pipe from the patient's arm.

It took a minute for the firefighter to respond because he couldn't stop laughing.

Our charge nurse once answered a phone call from a man who wanted to know how many pills to take to commit suicide. She said she could not legally tell him that, but the 911 operator would know and dispatch didn't have rules against giving callers that information.

The man called 911 and was brought in just a few minutes later for a mental health eval.

Banged Up

EMS responded to a single-vehicle MVA on the outskirts of town. The head medic called in report of a female, early-twenties, with bruising and lacerations to her face, head, and upper torso, as well as a broken nose and complaints of neck pain. We suspected the patient had swerved to miss a deer or had not seen a turnoff, given that it was after midnight.

When I went to the patient's room, she was every bit as banged up as the report that was called in. She had two black eyes, was receiving staples to a gash on her head, blood dripped down her face and bloodied her waitressing uniform, and she wore a neck brace.

"Hurry up and ask your questions," the doctor told me. He wasn't usually grumpy or demanding, but it was clear the night had gotten the best of him. "As soon as I get these last two staples in, she's going to CT."

I nodded. It didn't take long at all to verify the patient's information because she had been to the doctor's office a day prior, so all I had to do was make sure her information had been entered correctly at that visit.

"And where did this happen, again?" I asked.

"Over by the hog farm."

"Did you just lose control, or…?"

The patient snorted, then cried out in pain. She then laughed.

"Well, kind of. I was listening to this song and started headbanging, and—."

"Headbanging?" asked the doctor.

"Yeah," the patient replied. "You know, waving your head back and forth."

"I know what it is," answered the doctor. "You were doing that while you were driving?"

"Right up until I hit my head on the steering wheel."

The patient looked at me. "When I hit my head, I accidentally turned the wheel and hit a tree."

Her doctor stifled a chuckle and then shook his head in disbelief.

"The airbag went off and broke my nose," continued the patient. "And my neck hurts."

That was the first and only time I've ever met someone injured in a vehicular accident that was directly caused from headbanging. The patient was released with minor injuries.

A mom brought in her 12-year-old daughter for a pregnancy test. As I was registering the girl, she tried to remove her cell phone from the pocket of her skin-tight jeans and screamed. She broke her middle finger when it became stuck in her pocket.

Mom's response?

"Maybe if you didn't wear such tight pants, you wouldn't be in here to see if you're going to be a mama, either."

For Your Kindness

A frequent flyer was brought in for an overdose. It was the fourth overdose the hospital had handled in an hour, and we were only in the second hour of our twelve-hour shift.

Officers arrived and asked the patient if he was in possession of illegal substances, as if anyone in their right mind would answer 'yes' to that. Occasionally, officers would receive a positive answer, and they'd make an arrest, so I guess it was worth a shot to ask. The officers did not conduct a search of the patient, and they left the room so my coworker could have the patient sign consent forms.

When she emerged from the back, her eyes were wide and she was breathing heavily.

"What happened?" I asked. "What are you freaking out about?"

"He handed me a tiny baggie filled with drugs," she whispered.

"Who did?"

"The guy in three-B. He said it was a present for being so nice to him every time he comes in."

"Oh my God," I laughed. "What did you do?"

"I gave it to the cops! What did you think I was going to do with it? I've never even smoked pot."

"Maybe you should," I joked. "It calms you down."

"How do you know?"

"Uh, only because I use it all the time."

"You do?"

"No! I Googled it. Duh."

(That's the truth. I don't mess with drugs, unless you count wine. Lord knows I adore my wine.)

The girl went on a panicked rant for at least fifteen minutes, and then she was called to the nursing supervisor's office to give an official statement for hospital and police records.

My coworker never showed up for her shift the next day. One of the nurses knew her outside of work and told me she was afraid that the man would seek revenge against her, so she quit her job and ended up taking a job at a grocery store.

My new neighbor got drunk tonight and stole a live chicken out of someone's yard. He received a ticket, but no jail time, as he agreed to release the bird back to its owner. This isn't hospital-related in the slightest, but I think it goes to show that I'm a crazy-magnet.

What Would You Do for...?

Two unit clerks went home early, both stricken with the flu. This meant ICU, Inpatient Hospice, and Peds were without a clerk to push/call in orders to the pharmacy, Central Supply, or transfer patients from floors/beds. We had two registration clerks in the ER, so my coworker and I played 'rock/paper/scissors' to choose which of us would be playing float until the two floors could convince someone from day shift to come in early. We also knew we were really playing to see which of us would act as a float for the rest of our shift, because four inches of snow had blanketed the town in about three hours, and the snow plows were concentrating on the interstates first; they wouldn't touch the roads surrounding the hospital until the very last minute. I knew nobody would want to wake up early and want to deal with that.

"Just take it," my coworker begged on the third time we tied, both throwing down a closed fist.

The last time she'd been called upstairs, a 90-year-old man reached up and grabbed her breast.

"You take it."

I didn't have a story like hers. I just didn't want to go upstairs because I didn't like the ICU charge on duty. I can't believe that after nearly a decade, I still hold so much dislike for that woman.

"Take it, and I'll handle John Doe from start to finish for a week."

I thought about this offer. John Doe was a frequent flyer, as in a *daily, multiple visits per day* frequent flyer. It was rare that he wasn't intoxicated when he registered. He had a habit of flirting with all the women in the ER, and I couldn't recall the last time he'd been admitted to the ER that he didn't pull out his penis to show all the ladies. He babbled, too, so no conversation was ever quick. If you walked away too soon or tried to cut him off as he was speaking about something that didn't matter or didn't make sense, he'd become violent. We were instructed to basically talk to the man as long as it took for him to finish his stories. That rule came down from the self-proclaimed humanitarian, out-of-touch, 'it's a lie if you tell me you're ever too busy to take a break' ER director herself. She said Doe's violent behavior was avoidable and he was 'lashing out' because we were all offering poor and impolite human interaction.

"You have to talk to him after discharge, too," I said, "when he's waiting for his cab."

"That's kind of pushing it," my coworker said with a frown.

"You said start to finish. It's almost three, too. You'll have to check on patients up there. I bet that guy from the jail is up and ready to get a handful of boob. And he'll really want it, too, because it'll probably be the last he gets for a while."

"Fine," she reluctantly sighed.

"A week," I reminded her. "From the minute he walks in, till the time he leaves the grounds, he's gonna be all yours."

I told the nursing supervisor I'd act as float, and she told me to go to ICU first because the charge was throwing a fit because she 'wasn't paid to file charts.' As I rode up in the elevator, I mentally responded to every snotty thing she could possibly say to me while I was upstairs, just so I could get it out of my system and hopefully not say aloud what I was thinking.

Now, the hatred I had for this woman wasn't learned over time. It was a pretty immediate hatred, which I picked up within the first ten minutes of meeting the woman about a year back. She was just a miserable, hateful, rude woman, and I couldn't stand her.

"Kelsey, what took you so long? This is your job, you know."

"Kerry."

"Huh?"

"Kerry, not Kelsey."

We'd only met about five hundred times. Shame on me for expecting her to call me by my real name. In all fairness, I knew hers, too, but when I talked about her I chose one that I can't use in this book.

She rolled her eyes. "Okay, whatever." She pointed to a mess of paperwork on the desk. "Organize this. File it. Some, you'll have to put in the computer. I know registration is barely competent, but you can manage that, right? You start that."

I gave her the 'okay' symbol with my fingers.

"Don't start getting crappy with me. Just get over here and do it."

She turned, and I wanted to give her a middle finger salute, like a minute into being on her floor.

"Oh," she told me, turning to face me again, "No liquids for 433, 37, or 42. Eighteen, 21, and 37 also need bedpan assistance."

"You're down an aide, too?" I exclaimed.

"What?" she asked, copping a nastier attitude. "You're telling me you're not qualified enough to hand out water and help someone pee?"

Well, not for getting the pay of a secretary, I wasn't.

"I just didn't know you didn't have an aide, that's all. Nobody told me."

"I just did. Go do room checks. And stop standing around. I want those papers filed before you answer pages to any other floors."

In my head, I called that woman a few more names I'd missed in the elevator. Still, I went about my business and printed out a patient list. The first few patients on the list were either sound asleep on their own accord or were sedated. I helped two patients use the restroom and offered up water to several others. For a few seconds, I stopped to talk to the officer in the room at the end of the hall. His prisoner was sleeping, following the surgery to remove two bullets from his back.

On the other side of the hall, the patients were awake and demanding. I argued with a little old lady because she swore up and down that she was allowed to have solid foods, but her chart said no, and a nurse I tracked down confirmed that. I returned to the room and repeated to the patient that her chart read that she was not allowed to have solid foods. The woman threw a book at me. I marked her off my list and moved to the next patient.

"Well," he said to me as I entered, "you're not a nurse."

I looked down to my business casual outfit, back to him, and said, "No. No, I am not."

"That's okay," he replied with a light laugh. "You can still probably help me, right?"

"Maybe," I nodded. "I'm basically allowed to offer non-medical assistance. Just up here because someone got sick. I'm taking over her paperwork tonight."

"I don't need medical assistance." He nodded to his leads and IV, "They got me all covered there."

"Looks like it."

"Can you help me, though? See, they put my clothes someplace, and I need my coat. Got some stuff in my pockets I want."

"Not cigarettes, right?" I asked.

The older man shook his head. "Never been a smoker."

"Ah."

"Don't worry, no drugs or anything. I bet you see a lot of that kind of stuff in here."

"Sure do."

"Yeah, heard that man over there," he nodded across the hall, "whooping and hollering. Heard he robbed a liquor store and got shot up."

"I'm not quite sure what happened," I lied, though what the man heard was correct.

The man glanced around the room. "I really need my coat. I don't know where these people put the damn thing. Can you help me find it?"

I rummaged through the dresser drawers in the room and looked in the closet. In the end, I found it in the bathroom, hanging from the back doorknob.

I handed the man his coat just as the charge nurse angrily called out, "KELSEY!"

"I'll be right back," I said to the patient. "Just give me a second, and I'll be back to put your coat up."

"Okay."

The charge was in the hallway, pointing to the old woman's room. "Did you tell her she could eat?"

"No."

"Yes, you did! Everyone up here knows she's not allowed to have solid food. But, no, you come up here, and now the patient is upset. What is your problem?"

My pager beeped. It was a stat-page from Peds. The way the system was set up, the only people in the hospital that could change Peds orders had to use the floor computers.

"Don't you even think about leaving me with this mess, Kelsey."

"Peds has an emergency. I have to go."

"No. You're going to stay here, and you're going to go back in there and tell the patient that you're sorry, that you made a mistake and opened your mouth when you shouldn't have. And you're going to do it before she files a complaint with a patient advocate."

My pager beeped again. I couldn't stay there, and I didn't have time to argue. I rode the elevator down to Peds and pushed through a group of family members who huddled around the room that was located near the unit clerk area. Some were yelling, some were crying. Security guards, the nursing supervisor, and the charge nurse were all there, trying to move the family out of the way and stop two women from fighting.

A nurse approached me and told me to get the child transferred from Peds to the ER, and then someone from the ER (either the unit clerk in back or my coworker up front) would call the helicopter for transport to a Peds hospital a few hours away.

I transferred the patient and security yelled for me to call 911. I wasn't sure why, but it soon became apparent that the child was suffering from cancer and the biological parents were arguing with each other. In addition, the child's step-parents were arguing with each other. What started as a verbal attack soon became physical, and some of the child's family members were trying to keep staff from treating or transferring the patient.

The nursing supervisor sent me back to ICU to finish filing. One of the guards hollered at me to hold the elevator for them as the doors were closing, but it was too late.

When the doors opened to ICU, the charge nurse was standing in the hallway, with her hands up in the air. The two other nurses on the floor surrounded the male patient who'd asked for his coat earlier. That guy was unplugged from his monitors and was standing in the doorway of his room, still wearing his gown, with wires hanging off his body.

Oh, and he was waving a hunting knife around.

I remained in the elevator and it started moving back down to Peds. Two officers stepped inside. I turned my head and kind of shot them a look of bewilderment.

"So, uh, there's a guy on ICU, and he has a knife," I said.

"That's why I told you to hold the doors."

"I may have given him the knife."

"What? Why would you give a patient a weapon?"

I panicked. "I mean, I didn't *mean* to. He was looking for his coat, so I gave it to him and came down here."

"Did you see where he was? Was he saying he wanted anything? Was he screaming?"

I shook my head. "He wasn't saying anything. The nurses were telling him to calm down. He was standing in the doorway of his room."

"Young? Old?"

"Older. Like, maybe early-sixties."

"You talked to him?"

I nodded. "Yeah, like a few minutes ago. He was nice."

The other guard laughed. "Sounds that way."

I stepped off the elevator again as the guards approached the knife-waving patient. The nurses scattered.

"Kelsey gave him the knife, he said," the charge nurse told the guards.

"Kerry already told us," one responded.

The guards tried to get the patient to drop the knife, but he refused.

Finally, after about five minutes of threats of arresting the man, someone thought to ask, "What do you want?"

The man's answer was fairly simple: He'd been in the ICU for eight days for pancreatitis and complications. He was placed on a no-liquids, no solid foods diet. He was scheduled for a gall bladder removal surgery, but in that time, he contracted pneumonia, so that meant he couldn't have surgery, and he still couldn't eat. One doctor informed the man he could have broth, but another doctor came on duty and told the man he could not, that he'd have to continue nutrition through a tube, and following his gall bladder removal, the staff would *see* when and if he could tolerate foods without using the feeding tube. The man told security that he just wanted one of the doughnuts the nurses had at their work station.

It was a long rest of the shift. The charge nurse, up until the day she transferred to another local hospital, hated me. I can tell you with absolute certainty that the feeling was mutual, though I try to make it a point not to hate anyone. She is my exception. I didn't get in trouble for what happened because I honestly didn't know the man had a weapon in his coat, and I certainly had no idea he would go ballistic over a pastry.

Once upon a time, the cops were contracted as security for the hospital. One of the officers waited for a woman to come to the ER desk and asked her, "Have you maybe had a bit to drink tonight?"

She said no, but the wall she hit before placing her car in 'park' told a different story.

Professional Injury

A man carried a woman inside. She was unconscious and only wearing a bra and skimpy little panties. We tried to stop the man from leaving, but two petite registration women versus a portly, at-least-six-foot-tall man was no match. He hopped in his car and sped off, without any of us managing to write down his license plate number.

My coworker called the triage nurse, who took one look at the unconscious woman on the lobby floor, turned around, and ordered us to call the back for a bed and lift assist.

Surprisingly, few people seemed to be interested in this event. Most of the patients in the waiting room glanced over to the bystanders, but returned their attention to the television or their family members. I remember thinking that I wished it could always be that way, but we all know it that wish didn't pan out.

Security came down to the lobby and two officers asked us questions, most of which my coworker and I couldn't answer because we hadn't paid enough attention to the man as we paid to the patient.

We entered the scantily-clad woman in the system as a Jane Doe. RNs popped smelling salts, but the patient kept passing out. A scan showed she was experiencing a brain bleed, and the ER doctor did not feel comfortable in guessing if the woman would make it through the night. The triage nurse told my coworker that the woman's vital signs weren't looking great, and the back had tried to transfer the woman three times to Critical Care, but she went from stable to needing immediate intervention each time.

It was a sad case, really. We assumed the man who'd dropped her off beat her to the point of unconsciousness, panicked, and brought her to the ER. That scenario made sense.

Halfway through my shift, a woman and a man entered the lobby and both were glancing around, peeking in the waiting room and down the halls.

"Can I help you?" asked my coworker.

The woman looked to the man to answer. She was wearing a tight vinyl skirt and a mismatched cami top.

The man nudged her by poking his elbow against the center of her back and nodded for her to move forward.

"I'm looking for my friend. She was supposed to meet me after an…appointment."

I didn't realize I was staring at the man until he cussed at me.

"You know where she is, don't you?" he asked me.

"Who?" I asked.

"My girl. She's here, isn't she?"

The man started to go on a rant, referring to the woman as a female dog.

"If she pulled this [crap] again, trying to get out, I'll kill her. I swear to God, I'm done with her disrespecting me like this. I make sure she's paid. I make sure she doesn't go hungry. She wants a bump, I make sure she gets it. And then she wants to run away and cry about how she wants out? Nope. Nope."

The woman tried to calm the man down, but he pushed her and she fell. Security came out of their office and the man ran. I don't know if he thought the officers were unarmed guards or maybe he thought he could outrun them...I'm not quite sure what he was thinking, but when the city officer tackled and cuffed the man, that guy started apologize real quick.

The woman picked herself up and approached the front desk. She didn't seem to care about her, ahem, 'friend' getting arrested.

"Can you tell me if she's here? Her real name is Jane. Her work name is Joan."

We struggled with this because we didn't know (with facts) that this woman knew our patient. However, common sense said it was likely.

My coworker called the nursing supervisor and the decision was made to allow the woman at the desk to see the patient. Just as we thought, the woman at the desk identified the patient. She even gave us the location of the patient's 'appointment,' a practice the two women used as a failsafe, should one of them make an 'appointment' and not return.

Officers visited the location and witnesses at the motel offered up a name. The name on the room registration was fake, but the name on the credit card used to rent the room was real. By dawn, officers had a name and location for the man who'd left the woman in the ER lobby.

According to that man, he paid for sex while his wife and kids were out of town. He said that the patient was removing her stockings when her toe caught in the netting and she fell. She hit her head on the corner of the bathroom counter. The man stated he could not keep the patient awake, and he didn't want his wife to know he'd been with a sex professional, so he thought he'd just drop the patient with us and she could receive the care she needed. He argued that he should not be arrested because 1.) he paid for a service he did not receive, 2.) he did not cause bodily harm to the patient; he was simply acting as a good Samaritan by bringing her to the hospital.

The patient was eventually moved upstairs and was later transferred to another hospital for surgery. One of the nurses said the patient lived, but she required rehab after losing some of her motor functions. A few months later, I saw one of the officers sent out to find the man who'd dropped the patient at the ER. The officer said the woman could remember the entire incident and stated it happened just as her client had reported.

Patient's mother: "He was trying to jump on a waterbed and fell."

My 18-year-old coworker, after she registered the child: "What's a waterbed?"

When the Band
Comes Around

I was lucky, but not lucky enough.
Okay, maybe I should explain that better,
huh?

A popular (or it was back then, at
least…they may still have a decent
following) band came to the city. We were
dreading it, as in placing our names in a hat
to determine which lucky person(s) would
get the day(s) off. In the past, the band's
crowd wasn't so much of a problem for
police as it was for the ER. Years before,
we were dealing with obnoxious, drunk
and/or stoned college kids who thought
anyplace but an emesis bag or toilet was a
great place to puke or pee. I, for one, didn't
want to work any of the three nights the
band was back in town.

When the neutral party picker—a member of housekeeping—drew my name from security's ball cap not once, but twice, I was beyond relieved. I was disappointed that my name wasn't chosen a third time, but I was overall ecstatic that I would be scheduled off for two of the nights the band played.

I listened to the scanner on my days off. I should add that as I was listening, I was lying around in pajamas and sipping wine, occasionally chuckling at what my coworkers were faced with as I sat on my butt and didn't have a care in the world.

Karma came back and bit me hard on that third night.

I'd say we had a solid eight officers on standby in the ER, solely present to control any combative patients that would arrive. Additionally, three extra security guards were scheduled. The rest of the city police officers were split between 'normal' calls and calls pertaining to the band's crowd, which amounted to more than 15,000 people per day. During the first two nights, more than 100 arrests had been made and our ER numbers were nearly quadruple the average.

I can't even begin to count how many drug or alcohol-related patients we registered on that third night. One girl and her friend were handcuffed together, as in one handcuff was attached to one girl's wrist, while the other was attached to the other girl's wrist. Their friend brought them to the hospital because the girls were drunk and nobody had a key to the cuffs. An officer cussed under his breath as he freed the two barely-out-of-high-school girls. He told us he wasn't going to bother with charging the teens for underage consumption or being drunk in public because 'being stupid enough to handcuff yourself to another person [was] punishment enough.'

RNs were up to their ears in overdoses. At one point, we ran out of ER rooms and started seeing patients on the second floor. Goodness, it was a mess.

One particular person I recall was not a patient, though he probably should have been. This man accompanied his friends, both of whom were admitted for dangerously-high BACs. The man, probably in his early-twenties, was escorted from the ambulance bay and directed to the waiting room. A medic ordered the man FIVE times to sit down, but the man appeared too wired up to stay still.

As I registered new patients, I saw out of the corner of my eye that the man in the waiting room was behaving oddly. At one point, he stood on the chair and danced. A few moments later, he removed his shirt and shorts. One of our security guards entered the waiting room and told the man to put his clothes back on. The man then took to changing the television channel. He flipped through the fifty-something channels three times. He finally settled on QVC and sat on his knees, with his nose about two inches from the television screen.

"Do you—Hey, do you see this?" he shouted to other patients and families in the waiting room. He pointed to the television screen, at a shiny blouse up for sale. "That's a thing of beauty, huh?"

Then the man began speaking to the saleswoman on the screen.

"Isn't this just exquisite, ladies?" asked the host.

The man nodded. "Yes. That is *absolutely* exquisite. You would look *stunning* in that."

I giggled and wandered to the back to drop off paperwork.

When I came back to the front, the man wasn't in front of the television anymore. In fact, I couldn't see him in the waiting room at all.

A few minutes later, a mother carrying a toddler on her hip approached the registration desk.

She started with a sigh, and I was positive the next words out of her mouth were going to be asking how much longer it would take to be seen.

"Look," she hissed, "my kid's already sick, okay? She's been vomiting all day. Her fever was 102 before we left the house."

"I'm sorry," I replied. "We're moving as quickly as we can. It's just that there's a band in town, and with all the extra peo—."

She shook her head. "It's not that. Even if you guys saw her and gave her medicine right now, it'd still take a while to work. I work at a restaurant. I'm patient, don't worry."

"Well, thank you," I said, with a hint of confusion about why she was at the desk.

"I can't handle this guy, okay? He crawled over to me, so I moved. Then he followed me. Then I moved again. Now he's lying under my chair, and when I try to move, he slinks on the carpet like a snake. Please make him get away from me. He's scaring me and he's scaring my daughter."

I looked over to one of the security guards. "You're up, man."

He assured the woman that he would handle the problem.

"Sir," I heard him say, "is there a reason you're hiding under the chairs right now?"

I didn't hear a response, but I did hear the guard warn the man not to make him go back in there again, or the police would be sent up to handle the next complaint.

"Took care of it," the guard told me, as he returned to his standing position against the back wall.

More patients came and went. Some came in freely but left in handcuffs. Housekeeping practically moved in the lobby to stay on top of mopping up vomit and security moved to directing people to restrooms. One girl squatted in the pot of the fake palm tree that was in the corner.

"No!" the guard yelled. "Go to the bathroom!"

The girl started to cry. "I can't make it stop!"

Well, nice knowing you, fake tree. I guess the interior decorators never thought that the silk plant would be used as a restroom.

While that was going on, I saw the weird guy from the waiting room do some kind of secret agent barrel roll out of his chair and he rolled to the center of the room. When I looked directly at him, he appeared alarmed and did a somersault toward the television, one of those large, heavy televisions placed on a square table.

"Hey," I said to a police officer, as she passed by the registration desk. "Will you go in there and see what the hell that guy is doing?"

"Which one?" she asked.

"Oh, you'll know when you see him, trust me."

She didn't seem amused whatsoever. She walked over to the waiting room and the man flipped out. When he tried to somersault away from the television, he fell over and knocked the television off the table. We heard a loud pop from the waiting room and then there was a thin swirl of gray smoke that swiveled upward.

"Sir!" the officer yelled.

The man looked for a place to run, but the only way out meant he'd have to run by the officer. Instead, he tried to open one of the windows: a whole-wall window that is incapable of opening.

"Help!" the man yelled. "Help me! I'm trapped!"

"Sir, why are you shouting right now?"

"Because I sell acid and I'm carrying it in all my pockets," he shrieked wildly.

I started laughing so hard I thought I was going to puke.

The officer laughed, too, and asked, "Have you been dipping in your supply?"

Knowing it was over for him, the man once again removed his shirt and pants, turned around, and dropped to his knees. He then said, "Okay, I'm ready. You can shoot me now. I've said my goodbyes."

"Nobody's getting shot tonight," the officer laughed. "You are being placed under arrest, but I promise I won't discharge my weapon if you cooperate. Are you going to cooperate?"

The man began sobbing.

"I'm so sorry about the TV. I love TVs. I've owned them my whole life."

The officer was laughing so hard she had to call for help with the arrest.

By the time that band left town, I think the cops reported something like a million dollars in drugs were seized and about two hundred arrests were made.

Setting: 35-step staircase leading from the top floor to hospital roof

Character: Teenage boy, at hospital while mother visits boyfriend for heroin overdose

Plot: Despite being told he may *not* run up and down the stairs for 'exercise,' teen decides to do it, anyway

Climax: Teen trips, hits face on a stair, breaks three teeth; teen then rolls down stairs, hits head on railing

Conclusion: Call to emergency dentist, following 13 sutures to head

Knocked
Something Loose

A patient threatened to sue the hospital, which was a common threat in a large city. Registration usually took the brunt of these complaints, most commonly from patients recently discharged from the ER and unhappy with their treatment plan or what they often felt was a lack thereof.

This case, though…wow. Just wow.

A woman was transferred to the ER from a bathroom near HR. She was dressed to the nines: a black pencil skirt, stiletto heels, and an expensive pleated blouse. We were told she had an interview scheduled for the time she was admitted as a patient.

This woman was anything but pleasant. There are many names for the Devil: Satan, Lucifer, and sometimes the Beelzebub. On this day, we just called the Devil 'Jane.'

Our patient insisted upon recording her entire admission with her cell phone. She was rude and nasty. If someone asked her a question, she would reply snidely.

"Can you tell me where it hurts the most?" a nurse asked.

"Well, I fell, so where would you think it'd hurt the most?" the woman spat back.

This went on and on for some time. She showed no signs of stopping when registration entered her room for her to sign consent forms.

My coworker returned to the desk about thirty seconds after she'd disappeared into the patient's room. This young girl was in tears.

"I'll quit if you make me talk to her again," she told everyone at the front. "She said she was going to sue me and that I'd lose my job. I don't want to lose my job. I need the insurance."

I took the consent forms from my tearful coworker and went to the back.

"Ms. Smith," I greeted her, "I'm Kerry from registration."

"That'd still not be worth anything, even if I'd asked," said the woman. She kept her camera pointed at me and began adding commentary.

"You can see clearly that this person's nametag is difficult to read. She's not wearing business footwear. She should have her hair placed up to be around patients."

I waved to the camera and wanted to say, "I'm Kerry Hamm. Welcome to Jackass."

"Thankfully," I said instead, "our hospital administrators actively evaluate the employee handbook, and I am well within the proposed guidelines."

"This is being used in court," said the woman.

"Well, I'm glad I put on eyeliner today," I joked. "I'm a neutral party here," I explained seriously. "I'm just here to confirm and document your information. I need a few forms signed."

The woman shook her head. "I want a lawyer."

"You can call one, if you'd like, but I'm not getting involved."

"You've already broken policy. You're involved. Now, I want a lawyer."

"I can come back after you call and speak with your lawyer."

"I'm not signing anything. I'm not at fault here."

I refused to argue with the patient, and this made her even more frustrated. She spoke more commentary to the camera as I was leaving the room, saying things such as if the hospital really thought she was at fault, I would have tried harder to have her sign the consent forms or verify information. I bit my tongue to avoid turning around and telling her that there were nearly thirty other patients to speak with before they were discharged. I couldn't very well stand in this woman's room all day.

The woman's lawyer never showed. What a big surprise. The patient was discharged and was still recording when she left her room and entered the lobby. She approached the desk and demanded each of the registration clerks to look at the camera and say their full names and birthdates.

She cussed at me when it was my turn.

"I believe you already know me," I said, after she called me a derogatory name. "Please have your lawyer contact my employer, should you need anything else."

(By the way, I got in trouble for that line, for 'encouraging' a patient to seek litigation. It was a pretty big deal. I had to meet with three people from HR and then had to meet with something called a 'crisis' team, which I think was like a PR team for our facility. They gave me a list of approved things to say, should I ever have to deal with those types of threats in the future.)

None of us even knew why the patient was in the ER, except that she had fallen. I mean, that was, until she announced to everyone that she had been trying to flush the toilet with the toe of her shoe, when she fell and hit her head on the tile floor. She claimed the hospital was at fault for all of this because they did not prevent germs from being on the toilet handle, and she said the bathroom floor was 'too hard' and the facility should have known that injuries could occur, should someone fall while in the restroom.

Get this: after she announced this, she threatened to sue the hospital for releasing confidential elements of her injuries because the waiting room at this location was not separate from the registration area.

Triage called security at this point, which really brought out the crazy in this chick. She shouted and swung her $500 handbag at the guards and was completely off her rocker.

She was walked off the property, but later returned to threaten a lawsuit because she was denied a position with the hospital. We learned (from the woman) that she had applied as an ER registration clerk. HR confirmed this.

Good call on not hiring that nutjob!

Not Fit for Duty

On her first day in the ER, my coworker had been doing a fantastic job. She was sweet as honey and didn't mind vomit, so I was incredibly grateful that she registered ill patients at the desk and entered their rooms to have forms signed/ missing information filled in. Because it was winter, most of our patients had been pukers, so the girl had a long six hours. I did my fair share by completing and filing her paperwork, as well as picking up patients while she was in back and completing our office task list.

A father came in, holding a young boy. At first glance, the child's face appeared to be covered in blood. My coworker looked away for a moment and mumbled something.

"Are you okay?" I asked.

"Uh, yeah," she said, with a big smile. "Everything's fine."

The phone rang and I grabbed it.

"Can you get them registered?" I asked. "This is a transfer call and may take a minute."

The girl nodded.

As soon as she faced that father and child again, she started swaying and I thought she was going down. She grabbed her chair for leverage and eased to a seated position.

The father picked up right away on what was occurring.

"Oh," he said, "it's not blood. It's paint. It's okay. It's just paint."

My coworker chuckled nervously and the color came back to her cherub cheeks. "Oh, okay."

"Yeah," the father nodded. "I was out of the garage for a whole two seconds, and when I came back, he'd dumped a container of paint on his head."

"Oh! Wow."

The father then said, "Yeah, I yanked him away from the shelf as it was falling. That's how I got this."

He held up the side of his hand to show her a bleeding gash and then yanked his arm back, as if he'd forgotten he probably *shouldn't* have showed the girl.

My coworker's eyes rolled back and she fainted, right there in her chair.

"Jill," I said into the receiver, "I have to call you back in a minute. New girl just passed out."

Jill laughed and we hung up.

My coworker thought it would be best to ask for a transfer to our sister department, where she'd work in an office setting and only see patients for scheduling and insurance verification. My supervisor agreed.

03:00, request for emergency dentistry until the patient could make an appointment at 08:00

Reason:

"I was rubbing a vibrator over my sinuses to clear them out, but then I dropped it and it hit my teeth."

One front, lower tooth cracked. One front, lower tooth broken in half.

Vibrator: 1; Patient: 0.

Hold My Beer and Watch This

Out in the country, people do stupid things all the time. I'd go as far to say that the level of stupidity in the country is worse than that in a city, just because there are more ways to get severely injured in the country. After all, most of us have grown up with firearms, parents who've let us go off unattended into the woods for twelve hours, we learn to drive at a young age (farm equipment, ATVs, and even street-legal/ordinary cars), and we suffer from a general sense of 'bad things never happen around here.' Now, add all of those factors to near-poverty (ham and beans for four nights straight), boredom ("No, I'm not driving you 45-minutes away just to roller skate for 20 minutes."), and a vast openness to explore, and—TA DA!—you now have created a virtual theme park of danger, and

132

dang, does it look exciting when the only other options you have are whiskey and jail. (The best-worst ideas have those aspects, too!)

Mr. John Smith was old enough to know better—at least you would assume so, being that he was in his late-thirties. Sadly, his age didn't factor in whatsoever. He and his buddies lived nearly an hour from our town or any other town that had more than a few homes and maybe a small post office. There's nothing to do over that direction. During summer, some of the college and high school kids go out that way to drink around the bonfire. Hunters go out there during season to bag a few deer. Other than that, the fields are barren during off-season and filled with tall rows of corn at other times. There aren't a lot of homes that way, with ten or twenty houses located miles away from one another.

John Smith didn't own a swimming pool. Drought left the creek bone-dry. A felony for shooting an owl and a DUI that followed a few months later meant Mr. Smith wasn't allowed to be in possession of firearms, so he sold them to pay his court costs, and he was on probation, so he wasn't supposed to drink. He couldn't afford cable. He didn't have internet in his home. The internet on his phone only worked when it wanted. John was temporarily laid off from a nearby factory due to the company's supply and demand fluctuations. Poor John didn't even have the money to run his air conditioning, so his doublewide modular home was a heat box in the middle of July.

One night, John thought 'screw it,' I guess. His friends arrived at his house with a few cases of cheap beer, dirt bikes, and the 'best' worst idea in this county.

The best-laid, absolutely thought-out plan was to speed a dirt bike up the mound of soil next to John's half-a-car garage/shed, then make a sharp right and land on another pile of dirt just behind John's modular home. This would probably be possible to someone 1.) who was trained or with a great deal of experience with BMX, and 2.) if the men didn't all have BACs at *least* four times the legal limit.

One of John's friends went first. He traveled up the mound of dirt, jumped over the garage, and landed not so well between the garage and the modular. When I say not so well, I mean the rider landed before the bike did, and when the bike landed, it snapped the rider's leg.

Because the other men were drunk or wanted to prove *they* could pull it off (or both), they *left* the injured rider between the garage and the house and promised they'd take him to a hospital 'in a minute.'

Next up was friend 2/3. He was successful in his technique and bragged about it.

Friend 3/3 decided he wanted to drink another beer before his turn, so he passed to John.

Mr. Smith, per the other friends, was all talk beforehand, boasting about how he knew he could pull off the stunt.

His friend said John's last words before handing off his can of booze were, "Hold my beer and watch this."

That, my friends, is a sure sign someone's about to end up in the emergency room. Seriously, I'd say about 99-percent of people who utter those words will end up in a hospital within an hour.

John Smith mounted a bike and traveled up the dirt at rapid speed. Here's where he made his mistake: instead of slowing and turning the direction of the bike toward the second mound of dirt, Mr. Smith accelerated as he passed over the garage and missed his shot at turning safely.

I don't know the point in all of this that John realized he'd messed up. Maybe it was as the bike was descending toward the roof of his modular home. Or, more likely in my mind, it was just as the dirt bike was crashing through the modular's sun roof.

Mr. Smith landed his bike in his living room.

As if the initial crash was not enough of a punishment, the dirt bike continued to operate inside the home, while Mr. Smith laid passed out on the floor, under his broken television set and glass. The dirt bike zoomed into the kitchen area and took out not only Mr. Smith's dining table, but also the kitchen island. Its final resting place was against the now-smashed refrigerator door.

John's friends called an ambulance. Because they were in the country, country defined in this area as 'take the first gravel road off the blacktop, turn to the gravel road a few miles down, then take the dirt road over the dip in the creek,' the ambulance service brought John and his broken-legged bud in close to two hours after the initial call for help. By this time, John had come to. He was found to have sustained minor bruising, superficial lacerations, and a concussion. Other than that, he was fine…fine enough to go to jail for breaking the law and immediately failing the terms of his probation. I think the worst part of all of this was John said he didn't have medical *or* homeowner's insurance. I don't even know if homeowner's insurance would have covered that type of accident.

Incident in Aisle One

Our triage nurse was late for her shift one night, which had us all worried because she had never been late in sixteen years of her employment.

"Did you have car trouble?" I asked, when she walked inside.

She shook her head. "No. I stopped at the grocery store for carry-in stuff, and some guy saw the scrubs."

The nurse continued, "He followed me to the parking lot, pulled down his pants, and wanted to know if he should go get seen for the rash on his penis."

"What'd you say?"

"I told him if he didn't pull his pants up and get away from me, he wasn't going to have to worry for much longer because he wasn't going to have a penis left."

<u>Proven Wrong</u>

When I moved back to the Midwest, following my time on the coast, I thought I'd known all there was to know about this area. I'd spent most of my childhood growing up locally, walking the woods, taking shortcuts through cornfields, heading over to the neighbors' home three miles away to bring our wandering dog back home. As an adult, there wasn't too much more to learn about the place. Everyone here knows that drugs are an issue, though I must admit I didn't know just how prevalent drug addiction in the county is until I worked in the ER.

You may remember how I talked about someone picking up a skunk in that first book. I told you that people in this rural area generally know which animals to mess with and which to leave alone. We have coyotes, deer, raccoons, opossums, skunks, and stray animals that rarely pose a threat to human life, unless these animals are provoked and/or carry rabies. In and near waters, we have water moccasins, and brown recluse spiders are also another concern for the area, as both the snakes and spiders pack a nasty bite. Some people— mostly farmers—have sworn to have seen bobcats in the area, but nobody's ever been able to present proof of these sightings. Only one person, to my knowledge, has a permit to house exotic animals on his property, but his lions, tigers, and whatever other animal he's fostering for rescue centers at the time are always secured. I can only think back to one time that one of his animals were loose.

So, after knowing all that, I'm sure you could understand why I scoffed and laughed at a housekeeper after he ran inside in the middle of the night and screamed, "There's a bear out there!"

In fact, I wasn't the only person laughing at this middle-age man. Security jokingly asked if the man had offered the bear a picnic basket. A nurse wanted to know how much the housekeeper had to drink when he went outside to take his break.

"It's not funny," the man said sternly. "I'm not kidding. There's really a bear out there. It's just walking around the parking lot."

"Maybe it forgot where it parked," I suggested with a chuckle.

"Don't believe me?" he asked us. "Go out there. It was in row J. I saw it and ran inside."

"Uh-huh," security said.

"Go out there. There's a freaking bear out there, I swear."

I stood. "If I go out there and you have John jump out and scare me, I'm going to bring in all the dirt I can find and pour it on the lobby floor. Like, there will be so much dirt in here, you'll think you were outside."

He shook his head. "I'm not joking."

I poked the security guard in the shoulder. "Well, are you coming?"

He shook his head. "I'm not that gullible. There aren't bears around here. I've lived here all my life."

"Yeah," said the nurse. "We're too far away from their natural habitats."

I shrugged. "Fine. I'm going. If I get killed in the parking lot, make sure you guys tell the newspaper that I asked you to go with me and you wouldn't."

The guard groaned. "Fine, I'll go."

We walked outside and couldn't see much out of the ordinary. Across the street, there was a woman riding a bike. I'm pretty sure she was drunk because she wasn't going in a straight line.

Out in the parking lot, nothing looked out of place. One car had its headlights on, so the security guard told me to remember the plate number so he could go through the employee registry and see if the car belonged to one of our own.

We heard a scraping noise by a locked entrance down the lot and I nudged the guard.

"Do you think there's really a bear out here?" he whispered. "Where would it even come from? They don't live around here."

The scraping grew louder, and the guard pulled a flashlight from his utility belt. He scanned the faint beam of light over the section of darkness. We didn't see anything.

"What a waste," I groaned loudly. "I'm going back inside."

I guess because we weren't whispering anymore, the loudness of my words caught the attention of the black bear that was trying to get into someone's vehicle. The security guard and I both gasped and ran back inside.

This was mainly an uneventful story, with the long story short being: went outside, saw a bear, ran inside, called the police department. By the time the cops got to the hospital, the bear was long gone. The guy who fosters animals said all his animals were accounted for, so nobody who saw the bear knew where it came from or where it went, and the people who didn't see it never believed us, so we just stopped mentioning the sighting to avoid sounding psychotic.

When engaging in anal intercourse, lubrication is always a fantastic idea. I've met two patients in all my years who've engaged without proper lubrication. One ended up with three stitches. The other ended up with seven stitches. Both were sent home with an irrigation bottle and one of those inflatable round pillows that women use postpartum.

Shh

Usually, when patients visited the ER with a request to keep information from their family and friends, it was because the patient was participating in an extramarital affair, on drugs, was underage and pregnant, or something scandalous. That wasn't always the case, though.

A car was driving erratically on the interstate, speeding one minute and then slamming on the breaks the next. It was ahead of me, and I wasn't about to get out of that lane because my exit was coming up.

"Please don't let this person get off at my exit," I prayed aloud. "And if they do, make them turn the other direction, not the way I'm going."

Haven't we all had that prayer at least once during our travels?

My prayer didn't work. The car did take the exit I was taking, and it did turn in the direction I was going. By the time I realized we were both going to the ER parking lot, I had calmed down and my mood went from frustrated to concerned.

The car parked a few spaces away from where I had parked. As I was walking toward the building, I noted a woman was trying to exit her car, but she seemed to be in great pain.

"Stay here," I said. "I'll bring a wheelchair. What happened?"

She looked me up and down. "I'm not telling a random stranger in the parking lot."

"I work here," I explained. "If you were in an accident, I can tell the nurses and see if we can get you back sooner."

"I fell," she said, so embarrassed that she had to look away.

She was babying her right ankle. The leg of her sweatpants, where the cuff wrapped around her ankle, seemed swollen, but I couldn't tell if that was due to her injury or the fabric.

"Do you hurt anywhere else?" I asked. "Did you hit your head?"

"No. I just fell and now my ankle hurts."

I nodded. "Just stay right here. I'll bring a wheelchair, and we'll get you inside for registration."

Once I explained to my coworkers what was occurring outside, I met the woman with a wheelchair. She was grateful, but worried.

"What all do you need for this?" she asked.

"Someone at the window or counter will ask for your identification later on. We'll start with your name, birthday, and your doctor or nurse practitioner. We'll ask for your allergies and little things like that."

"Can I use a fake name?"

I hesitated. "Uh, not really, no. I mean, if it's a matter of cost, we have departments that can work with you on—."

"It's not," she interrupted. "I just don't want my husband knowing why I'm here. If they send him the bill, he's gonna know, and then I'll be in trouble."

A red flag sprung up in my head. "Ma'am, if you are afraid of your husband, we can remove you from our directory. I can even call a counselor from a women's outreach program, if you'd like. Or, you can speak to any nurse in the back, and they can help you."

She seemed confused at first, but then she burst into laughter.

"My husband doesn't beat me," she said. "He just can't know I'm here because I told him the puppy wouldn't potty in the house, but she peed and I slipped in it. I had to drive myself because he said if she had an accident in the house, he'd get rid of her."

Our patient broke her ankle when she fell. We told her we would simply place 'fall' as her chief complaint, and the back placed a non-specified 'fall' in her chart, leaving out her story at her pleas. She said she'd waited 10 years to get a puppy, and none of us were about to ruin that for her.

Speaking of possible domestic abuse, we thought a frequent flyer lied about her constant injuries because her story was always, "I walked into a door," or "I tripped over a shoe."

She was leaving the ER after sutures to her lip, when she ran into a pole and busted her nose open. She said she didn't know it was that close to her.

It was at that point that a doctor suggested prescription glasses to the patient. She really *had* sustained injuries on her own, because she couldn't see properly! After getting glasses, she only came back once, and that was for a sports injury.

I still don't know how she drove without wrecking.

<u>Mr. Fix It</u>

One of the last patients I registered during my time as a registration clerk was still unconscious at the time of arrival. He was transferred to the ER by ambulance. His wife arrived shortly after his arrival and was probably one of the calmest family members I'd ever met.

After she gave me her husband's information, I said to her, "Give me one second, and I'll see if you can go back."

She flicked her wrist and said with a shake of her head, "Take all the time you need. I'm really in no hurry."

Perplexed by this, I asked jokingly, "Been through this before?"

She rolled her eyes and said, "Usually, he snaps out of it. This is only about the nineteenth time he's knocked himself out. I told him to stop trying to fix stuff around the house, but he won't admit he can't do it, and he won't pay for a contractor to come out when we need stuff fixed."

"What was he trying to fix?" I asked.

"He was trying to change the doorknobs," she answered. "He pulled on the old knob, and knocked himself out when it came flying out."

I chuckled. "No, really. What was he trying to fix?"

She popped her eyes at me. "The doorknobs. He literally knocked himself out while changing the doorknobs. Well, trying to change them, anyway."

"Maybe he'll call a handyman this time," I thought aloud.

She shook her head. "Doesn't have to. I finished replacing them before I drove here. I swear, this man breaks more stuff when he tries to fix it."

The wife went to the back eventually, and the registration clerks saw on the man's chart that he had been in the ER more than ten times over the course of the year for chief complaints such as: 'fell off roof,' 'nail punctured palm,' 'dropped hammer on foot,'

and 'hit self in face with piece of wood,
LOC (loss of consciousness).'

Overheard on scanner during St. Patrick's Day:

"Please respond to intersection of A and B. Multiple callers are stating a man is hugging a light post and crying loudly."

Foreign Bodies

Here's a list of all FB (foreign bodies) in ears and noses I can recall registering over my years:

* Please keep in mind that this list was not compiled with only minor patients in mind. Adults of sound mind are on this list, as well.

- Orange seeds and cherry pits
- *Hot Wheels* parts
- Rice
- Coffee beans
- Condom
- Peas
- Popcorn and kernels
- Pet food
- Illegal drugs
- Crayons and crayon pieces
- Gum

- Balloons (most typically water balloons or small, thin varieties)
- Legos
- Barbie shoes
- Pen caps
- A tooth (the boy apparently thought the safest place to keep his recently-pulled tooth was his left nostril)
- Batteries
- Buttons
- Noodles
- Yarn
- French Fries
- Rocks
- Silly Putty
- Modeling clay
- Jewelry (including a bracelet that had traveled through the nose and was extracted through the child's mouth)
- Grapes
- A nipple to a pet baby bottle
- A flower (a man was trying to show off by running a rose through his nose piercing, when the stem caught)
- Oil-filled jelly bath beads

Stunt Man

If you're unfamiliar with the sport called Parkour, it is basically trying to get from Point A to Point B in a complex and fast manner, but without assistance from ladders or equipment. Think about those stunt people in movies, the ones who can run up a wall or jump from building to building.

Maybe you think it's cool. I used to think that, too. I can no longer watch these videos, though, because every athlete has to start somewhere. Rarely, and I mean rarely, is someone born with this innate ability to perform at his/her highest ability and safely.

Imagine learning Parkour. Imagine running toward a wall and running halfway up said wall, while your body is in a position that is left unsupported. The greats have no trouble rapidly pulling off these stunts, seemingly working faster than gravity has a chance to work. But if you're a beginner, you're definitely going to have a bad time.

A Parkour beginner was brought in via ambulance one night and looked like someone had taken a metal stick to his face and upper torso. He had attempted to leap from one building to another, but he didn't quite make it. When I say he didn't quite make it, I mean he landed on his chest and face.

The young man lost most of his teeth during impact. Some, he swallowed. Others were in pieces on the ground. The man broke his nose, fractured his eye sockets, broke his jaw, cracked his skull, and cracked his sternum. He presented with cardiac arrhythmia due to the force dealt to his chest.

What was worst about all of this was that the man was conscious when he was brought in the ER. He couldn't speak, and he couldn't manage to produce tears, but he was extremely vocal during the transport. A doctor ordered medicine that would knock the patient out.

This young man had to go through multiple reconstructive surgeries and never quite looked the same again. Though he was on his parents' insurance, only a portion of his ER bill was covered. He was in the hospital for weeks.

The thing I find strangest about this case was that the man did not let the accident stop him. He figured he'd already experienced the worst thing that could happen in the sport, so he continued onward. I don't know if that's determination or utter insanity.

Big Brawl in the City

It's not every day you see a group of body builders carry in a friend, so when that happened, my coworkers and I stopped what we were doing and called for triage. The patient was bleeding profusely. One of the security guards held out his arms to keep incoming patients from tracking through the blood, but it was a holiday weekend and our numbers were through the roof. Like the small-town folks, the inner-city patients didn't seem to care much about if someone was bleeding to death or not. In fact, I think some of these people thought all that blood was a good sign.

'Maybe if he dies, I'll get taken back soon,' was probably a thought that crossed these peoples' minds.

"One of you call the back right now," ordered a flustered triage nurse. She tried to slip her hands in gloves but kept getting her fingers stuck. "And someone get me a pair of gloves. I swear, the next person who shoves a set of smalls back in the medium box, I'm going to just start beating you and probably never stop."

The patient was being held up by four friends. Two males held each of the patient's legs, while another held his upper body. A fourth man pressed a folded beach towel to the man's wound, but the towel was soaked and the blood showed no sign of stopping. Thankfully, the men seemed to have a handle on the situation. Though a bit shaky, they did not appear to be panicking.

"What happened?" the triage nurse asked.

All four men started talking at once.

"Can we please hurry it up here?" another male asked from the lobby. "I'm supposed to pick up dry cleaning in fifteen minutes."

"Feel free to leave," said the triage nurse, while the four men were working out who'd be the one to speak. "It's definitely going to be longer than fifteen minutes."

"I can't leave because my finger still hurts. I've been waiting out here for an hour. Now this is happening, and let me guess: you're going to take this idiot back before you take the people who've been waiting out here for all this time, right? This place is freaking ridiculous. Someone stupid comes in, and I end up having to pay for it."

Three of the men holding the patient turned to berate the man dressed in business attire. It was hard to hear anything over the sound of the patient's three friends arguing and threatening that man (and the man yelling back in return things like, "I'm not scared of you steroid freaks!"), and hear what the fourth friend was telling the triage nurse.

"How the heck do you hit yourself in the head with a sledge hammer?" the nurse exclaimed.

Well, I sure heard that.

Before I knew it, the man holding the bloodied towel against his friend's head dropped the thing and plowed into the man dressed in a suit and tie, knocking the man to the lobby floor and through a puddle of blood. The business professional didn't stand a chance against the bodybuilder. If I had to pick something for you to visualize, hmm…Let's say Mr. Burns from The Simpsons picked a fight with The Incredible Hulk—The Hulk from the updated movies, not the old television show, because the guy who was throwing all the punches was a lot more beefed up than Lou Ferrigno was required to be for his role.

Security tried to drag Mr. Beefy from Mr. Burns, but that wasn't working. When Mr. Beefy took a swing at one of the guards, his friends placed the patient on the floor and tried to keep their friend from fighting with the guards. Somehow, this resulted in the other three friends fighting with the guards and Mr. Burns. The injured patient was squirting blood all over the place and triage was yelling at registration to get help.

"I told you to call the back!"

162

"I did!" shouted my new coworker.

"If you did, there'd be help. You need to do what I tell you and stop screwing around."

"Well, maybe since you can just snap your fingers and get crap done, you should just call them yourself."

This is why I haven't told this story before. For starters, it did occur in the inner city, but the primary reasoning behind keeping mum is based on the intense staff on staff feud that I'm telling you about right now. It was embarrassing and unprofessional, really.

"You know what, Jane? You've been here two days and I'm already sick of your attitude."

"The feeling's mutual, honey."

"Stop," I said to the new woman. "Just stop."

"Oh, so you're on her side?"

"I'm not on anyone's side right now," I explained. "But arguing isn't going to help."

The new woman continued to argue with me as I picked up the phone and made another call to the back.

"I said we'd be up there in a minute, geez," answered the charge nurse. He sounded huffier than usual.

My coworker and triage were back to screaming at one another, and at least one guard and one friend from the Beefy-Burns-Security brawl were bleeding.

"We don't have a minute," I blurted out.

"Well, I don't have any beds."

"This guy is bleeding, like, *really* bad, triage is fighting with the new girl, and there's a massive fight going on. We need a bed or a place to put him or something. It looks like *American Psycho* up here. Even if you can't get a bed, we need help up here, like, right now."

"Is that what all that screaming is?"

"Yeah," I replied. "Don't send anyone small."

I hung up before the charge nurse had a chance to say more, and I dialed switchboard.

"Need you to call 911 and activate a code," I said.

"Which code?"

I hesitated because I couldn't remember the numerical codes or their designated colors.

"Uh...Well, the one where you call 911 for a fight and then the one where there's blood all over for stat cleaning and then the one where you call for big guys from other floors to come to this department and help us."

"Oh my."

"I don't know the numbers!" I shrieked, as one of the security guards popped the bleeding patient's friend in the leg with his night stick.

"Kerry?"

"What?" I shouted. "I'm freaking out. I don't know what you want from me. I don't know what I'm supposed to do right now."

"Kerry," she said calmly, "I can't do anything until you hang up."

Thank God all those women at the switchboard can keep it together when the rest of us can't. I don't know where we'd all be without our operators. Seriously, if you work at a hospital or facility where you have switchboard operators, treat those ladies with respect because they're going to be the ones saving your butts when crap hits the fan.

I slammed that phone down in its cradle and stood behind the desk, unsure of what to do next. Garbled words echoed through the PA system. My coworker slapped a pencil cup to the lobby floor in anger and the triage nurse was still screaming as she applied pressure to the patient's head. The fight to our right wasn't going any better. Other patients from the waiting area had joined in, making more victims than peace. Doors opened behind us and to the left of us. I thought this meant nurses from the back would be coming out, but it turned out the traffic was a group of discharged patients and family members.

"Go back," I shouted. "Don't come out here."

"Where do you want us to go?" a woman snapped. "I parked in the first row. I'm not walking all the way around the hospital, not with a kidney stone."

"You can't come out here," I hollered.

"I can do whatever I damn well please, missy."

The woman and her family members tracked through blood and then two of them doubled back to the desk to complain about it.

"This is unsanitary," one of the woman's adult daughters griped.

"I told you not to come out here." I pointed to the triage room. "Go back there and we'll fill out claims forms in a few minutes. It'll take care of the cost of your shoes."

"I've been exposed to human blood," the discharged patient growled. "I could get this whole place shut down."

"Would you two shut up and get in the car already?" the woman's husband shouted from the exit. "She told us not to come this way. We did anyway. Just wash your shoes off at home. We've been here four hours already. I'm hungry."

Thank God for that man being the voice of reason, because I didn't want to argue with the patient or her family.

"Kerry," the triage nurse yelled at me. "Did you call the back?"

I nodded. "John said they were out of beds. I told him to just find any place to put this guy and send help right away."

"That's how you do your job," the nurse said to my coworker.

"If she knew how to do her job, then there'd be someone up here, right?"

"Hey now," I said to the woman.

"I knew it. I knew you were on her side."

"There are no sides! What's with you and sides? Just stop arguing and sit down or something."

"You sit down. You've been telling me what to do since I got here."

"She's been telling you what to do since you got here," the nurse snapped, "and you still screw it up."

"Because I'm *training* you," I retorted.

Great. Now I was arguing, and it became a bickering triangle.

I shook my head. "I'm going to get help. The police should be here any minute."

"You called the police?" my coworker asked. "Security told me not to call the police, to call them. How do you expect me to learn all these stupid rules when you're here breaking them?"

I tried not to be rude, but at that point, I lost it. I pointed to the corner. "Hey, what's that, over there? Oh, that's right, those are our ER security guards, trying to break up…" I counted. There were a lot more people in that fight now than when it started. Holy crap.

I continued, "…Eight people. What am I supposed to do, get pompoms and cheer them on? Make a sign that says 'Go Security!' and hold it up for moral freaking support? But if you want to call security, be my guest. Oh, they won't answer you, though, because they're right over in that corner. So dumb!"

The charge nurse—a tall, strong ex-football player—came to the front with three orderlies, two male nurses from Radiology, and three guys from Peds, ICU, and Rehab. The charge nurse probably could have gotten involved in the brawl, but he held back the three orderlies to assist him and the triage nurse with the patient.

"Doors," he called to the registration desk in a strained voice, as he and the team struggled to keep the patient lifted. "Get the doors."

My coworker looked around helplessly. I ran over to where she was standing and hit the button on the counter that opened the double doors to a hall of fast track rooms. It would have to do, even though the fast track rooms were only equipped with one of those paper-covered tables you see when you visit doctor's offices. Some of the rooms didn't have chairs for family members to sit. I don't even think the patient could have fit on one of the tables in the fast track rooms, but no other rooms were available in our department.

One of the orderlies sprinted back from that area and called out from the doors as they were closing, "ICU gurney and call a trauma, high level-stat. Page surgeons now."

Three orders were there, they were all top priority, and I was training someone who didn't know how to do any of it. She didn't even know what any of it meant. I swatted the air to knock her questions about everything out of the air and told her I'd explain later.

"Go to the triage room and call switchboard. Tell Joan to call a stat Trauma Blue."

"I don't know what that means."

"She does. Call her. Now."

While she was calling the operator, I was logging on our web-page system that sent out a page to our surgeons. I also had the desk phone pressed against my ear and was waiting impatiently for someone from ICU to answer.

Finally.

"Hey Wanda, it's Kerry. We need someone to bring down a bed right away. We're out and we have a critical bleeder."

Wanda didn't argue, and we had the bed in fewer than three minutes.

I went to find my coworker. She was just standing by the triage phone, picking at her peeling fingernail polish.

"I didn't hear the code called."

"I can't do something like that unless I know what it is."

"Are you freaking kidding me?" I shouted. I shooed her away. "Go out there and wait for housekeeping and the cops."

"Operator?"

"Trauma Blue stat," I said, much calmer than the last time I'd phoned switchboard.

"Coming right up."

Housekeeping and the police arrived at virtually the same time. Neither appeared too pleased with the lobby scene. Multiple officers yanked brawlers from one another, started handcuffing people, and sat them in a line in the foyer. Most of the fighters were covered in blood they'd either sustained during the fight or picked up from the floor. Man, nobody in the back would like this.

In all of the madness, I'd forgotten to call the Nursing Supervisor, something I'd ordinarily do when things were out of control. I didn't even think about it until I saw her stomping down the hall.

"What in God's name is going on down here?" she asked me.

"Look," my coworker said, unaware of the supervisor's identity, "you and everyone else need to just lay off us, okay? We're doing the best we can. This is wild."

Even now, I can't describe the fear and embarrassment I felt for my coworker. My eyes were stretched open as far as they'd go. My mouth was agape. My heart was numb from shock.

The supervisor shook her head. She didn't have time to start in on the new woman.

"They're flying that man out," the supervisor told me. "So I need you to get some information from whomever has it, and then set up the flight."

173

I nodded.

"I," she said, "will help the unit clerk get all these people registered and to the decon showers." She pointed to the line of people in handcuffs.

I nodded again.

"And what do I do?" asked my coworker. "I can't register people yet."

"Just stand at the desk," I told her. "If someone comes in and they're not having chest pains or bleeding as bad as that guy was, tell them to park it and someone will be with them shortly."

The bleeding patient was transferred to a trauma center about two hours from our hospital. I still don't know exactly how he sustained his injury, but I do know the nurses and doctors were talking about how the man's brain was visible. I don't know what happened after he was transferred out.

Two of the patient's friends were arrested for the brawl, but charges were eventually dismissed. Mr. Beefy broke his hand in the fight and Mr. Burns had to get a few stitches. Three other patients from the waiting room who'd jumped in were treated for minor lacerations and were released. One of those three went to jail, but only because the officers ran his name and discovered he was wanted for an outstanding warrant. Our security guards were sent home early; one was bruised pretty badly, but the other didn't seem to have much wrong with him, other than a complaint of soreness. Their relief, two guards called in on their days off, were not happy to be at work. Our housekeeping members were equally unhappy. They spent an hour cleaning the lobby, and right after they finished, someone brought in a kid and the little girl puked all over the floor.

As for the triage nurse, my coworker, and myself…Well, the triage nurse and I were given verbal warnings but largely released on forgiveness related to the stress factor. My coworker was terminated at the meeting that took place the next day, with our boss citing that the woman did not act professionally and was mostly being dismissed for knocking the pencil cup off the counter space, but largely in part to refusing to call a code when she was directed. I didn't mean to rat her out, but the facts came out in the reports we each had to write up regarding the incident.

I still feel embarrassed regarding this incident because it's not the way any of us were trained, nor does it reflect the kindness we showed to our patients and to one another.

911 dispatch to EMS:

"Respond to report of female stuck to chain link fence. Patient reportedly pierced her genitalia on fence and cannot remove fencing. Officers on scene, following foot pursuit."

I Didn't Even Ask

One of the dumbest things I witnessed in the emergency room happened on a weekend when fraternities and sororities at the local colleges were running their pledges ragged. We'd already seen a handful of young kids in for things like alcohol poisoning.

A group of college girls brought in fresh meat. This girl had been crying, but had since stopped and was actively concentrating on breathing through her nose to prevent herself from crying again.

"I don't even want to know," I said to the girls, sure they were about to explain.

I registered the patient with a complaint of 'bottle stuck in mouth.'

Yep. This college girl had what appeared to be a bottle with a circumference slightly smaller than a Mason jar stuck in her wide-open mouth. The girls stated they tried 'everything' to remove it, short of breaking the glass.

Three doctors worked on removing the jar, but they finally had to dislocate the girl's jaw to remove the bottle. We all knew when it happened because the girl squealed for a minute and then passed out.

You know what? I still don't want to know why she did that. I do hope she learned from that incident. And, for going through all that embarrassment and pain, I sure hope she was accepted into that sorority.

My coworker once registered an older gentleman for a psychiatric eval at his request. He pleaded to be admitted because he said the only show his wife would allow to be viewed in the home was the 700 Club. He said if we didn't admit him, he'd go home and hang himself. He was admitted and he refused his wife visitation during his stay.

Devil's Music

Mr. Y had Alzheimer's and couldn't remember his family, his past, and he didn't recognize himself in the mirror. It was difficult to see the patient this way. He was essentially living in a stranger's body. Aides at his nursing home had tried using music from his younger days as therapy, as this method has been proven to help patients suffering from memory loss remember portions of their lives. Unfortunately, for Mr. Y, this didn't work. The nursing home said his family stopped visiting because Mr. Y didn't take kindly to strangers. In fact, when he came to the ER, it was the same routine: he kicked, screamed, spit, hit...He truly grew into that grumpy old man stereotype. He was meaner than a cat in a bathtub. If you could make it out of the room without being called a derogatory name, someone needed to get you a gold star. Mr. Y was downright hateful.

Someone from lab went in as I was waiting in the corner for Mr. Y to sign papers one night, and during her time in the room for routine labs, she was listening to her iPod. Mr. Y grabbed her wrist, so I poked my head out and called for a nurse. The nurse entered the room and scolded the tech for the unprofessional behavior, so the tech removed the earbuds from her ears and let them rest around her neck. She did not turn down the music, so it was blasting loudly.

Mr. Y cocked his head, raised his eyebrows, and asked the tech, "Jane, are you still listening to that Devil's music? What did your momma and I teach you. Dang, girl, you've put on some weight."

I giggled, while the tech frowned. The nurse seemed to be unsure whether to be concerned or amused.

"All this Fozzie Osborne and KISS and heavy metal," Mr. Y griped. "Girl, we tried to raise you right."

"My name is Jill, Mr. Y. I'm not Jane."

"You're not my daughter?" he asked. "You look just like her. Just more fluff in the middle."

The patient's nurse transferred the information of a breakthrough to the nursing home and we heard Mr. Y was started on another round of music therapy...using the music his 'rebellious' daughter listened to as she was growing up in her parents' home that believed in the calming tunes of Sonny & Cher and The Partridge Family. Mr. Y, according to what we heard from the nursing home, only seemed to respond to that 'heavy metal' music, and while he was listening to it, he could identify his family through pictures and could recall memories from his life. Most of them, we heard, revolved around his daughter sneaking out or getting caught smoking cigarettes.

Mr. Y came to visit us a few more times and always came to the ER with a cheap MP3 player, fully loaded with that 'Devil's music.' He stopped reacting violently toward staff, and his family even came to visit him a few times before he passed away.

Real Life in the ER

Working in the emergency room is reacting to repetition as you've never seen it before because you haven't, not with *this* patient. You saw all there was to see, heard all the complaints, went through the ropes with *that* patient. But *this* patient, she's never experienced chest pain before and she's scared. She's twenty or thirty or sixty and suddenly everything she's never finished in her life is haunting her. As she's standing before you, she wonders how her husband will find his wallet at three in the morning, how her daughter will learn how to apply foundation, how her three cats and poodle will react if she doesn't come home. *That* patient is different than *this* patient.

In the emergency room, you become a master at observation. You know your patient's grandmother is fighting back tears by the simple twitch of the old woman's nose, know mom is panicking through the smile on her face because she repeatedly grinds the base of her heart-shaped pendant over the thin silver chain around her neck. You know how to comfort everyone around you, know when to comfort everyone around you. You know when to offer coffee or when to ask if a patient's family wants to walk with you outside. You know when to pray. You know when to let that husband blow off steam, so you just walk away. Yet, when it comes to yourself, you can't predict when you'll burst into tears in the hallway or nurse's lounge or bathroom, and you don't know what could possibly ease this pain after losing a three-year-old to drowning or a 94-year-old to cancer.

You know stress if you work in the emergency room. You know how it feels to have someone breathing down your neck. You know the overwhelming sensation of every nerve in your body firing off when someone's demanding of you. Results aren't instant, your answer is dependent on the course of another person's actions, and you legally cannot offer more pain medication. Nothing is *right now* until there is a crisis. Then, everything is *right now*. There's never an in between.

When you work in the emergency room, you know the lewdest of sex acts by their street names, have been cussed out by hundreds of patients over the course of your employment, have humor blacker than a solid night sky, and yet the worst bad words you know start with 'Q' and 'S.' You'd rather have someone call you a whore than say, "It sure is quiet around here."

You gain appreciation for the little things in life after your time in the emergency room. You're more ready to forgive your toddler for drawing on the wall with a permanent marker because nothing is more permanent than the heartache of losing a child. Sleep becomes a luxury, and usually one you find you can't afford. When someone is in front of you in the grocery line, complaining about a twenty-cent coupon, you can appreciate that you have experienced far worse, and therefore, your nerves are steel in comparison to those around you. There's nothing you can't handle. There's nothing you haven't seen. There's nothing you can't get through.

It doesn't matter if you are a lab tech, x-ray tech, CNA, RN, LPN, MD, NP, housekeeper, Chaplin, secretary, security guard, or financial assistance advisor. When you can hardly make out the words, "Where is the bathroom?" through someone's sobbing, when you don't stop that man from throwing a punch at a brick wall because his kid is sick, when you panic because all 10 things in front of you are the number one priority, when you're overwhelmed because you only have two hands, when you're on your feet for nine hours, when you can't find two seconds to use the restroom, when you've never seen so much blood in your life…The emergency room becomes part of who you are, how you face life, how you face death. You can retire. You can quit. You can get fired. What you can't do is forget. You can't flick away what you've seen, the sound of a wife crying out after learning of her husband's death, can't shake the smell of a burn victim, rid yourself of the fears that encompass that place. You don't have to save lives to be bound to the ER. You don't need certification to see Mr. Y in your dreams or think of Mrs. Z when you pick up on a stranger's perfume.

So, to all of you—to the medics, police officers, hospital staff—hats off to you for living every single day, teetering between 'I love my job,' and 'I'm going to call in dead and flee to Mexico so I don't have to go back ever again.' You are appreciated. You are respected. It may not feel like the world is grateful to you, but it is. Thank you for your selflessness, for your dedication, for your kind hearts, for your ability to use humor to deflect stress, and for going back to do it all over again, even though you don't think you have it in you.

Now, it doesn't work in the *patient's* favor to do something stupid, but that stupidity is what keeps millions of people around the world with job security. So, by all means, if you want to drive your go-kart off a cliff to see if you can nail the landing, just make sure you have someone on standby to call 911.

A Message to Readers

If you do not follow my Twitter or Facebook accounts, I would like to take this opportunity to inform you that this is the final volume of '*Real Stories from a Small-Town ER.*' I have every intention to continue releasing books comprised of reader submissions. Unfortunately, all good things must come to an end, and such is the case with my personal stories.

This book wasn't difficult to write, but it was difficult to decide to write it. Most of these stories did not make the cut for previous volumes because they occurred in the inner-city. Some that I retold from my rural ER days, quite honestly, I didn't care for that much. I have omitted stories that I felt/feel would not be acceptable for a comedy/drama series. If you've read my books, you know a story has to be *horrific* to be omitted by such standards.

190

Since leaving the hospital scene, I can tell you straight up that the sky seems brighter and full moons no longer leave my stomach in knots. After years of ER registration, someone could cuss me out and I probably wouldn't even blink because there's nothing I haven't heard before. I gained patience over the years and have learned when to stress out and when to let it slide. I miss my coworkers tremendously and often miss assisting patients, but as I've ventured out again, I have had the 'pleasure' of seeing several patients. I'll say most of them are just as, well…they present in the rest of the world as they did/do in the emergency room. There are several kind patients I have been able to see since I left the hospital, and I am always glad to see these people because they seem so happy when they're not sick or injured.

Once again, I would like to thank you all for your interest in my series. I know you have options, yet you've chosen to read my books. I highly enjoy 'speaking' with readers through Twitter and Facebook. One reader messaged me and told me she reads my series to her mother, a retired nurse. Hearing that has been one of the most exciting moments of my writing career. I'm overjoyed to hear how these oddball, almost-unbelievable recollections bring people together. I know I have been blessed with a fantastic audience, and you will never know just how grateful I am for you. You have given me hope for the future and have allowed me to vent about frustrations that are now in my past, and trust me, it's greatly appreciated. I wouldn't be where I am today without your support and kindness.

When I am not sifting through reader submissions or pecking away at these medical comedies, I am actively working on several other books. I find medical comedies much easier to work on, so I know I can hop on over to this genre when my brain refuses to cooperate with young adult novels, adult suspense, or horror. I have five files open at this time, and I basically write what's in my head and then jump to the next file to do the same. One of these days, I hope anyway, I'll release a 'real' novel. Self-doubt is the killer of all dreams, and it stabs at me every now and then.

I want to note from a few reviews, that yes, I prefer to keep my medical comedies sarcastic and in plain-language. This isn't Pulitzer material, folks. I want my books to read exactly how I'd excitedly tell you the story if you were sitting next to me. I hope you've enjoyed them so far, and I do hope the humor translates correctly through the text.

For those of you who'd inquired, I did create a website. It's under construction, but I will continue to brainstorm about what to put on it. If you want to see something specific, please let me know and I'll see what I can do. I do my best to respond to every comment or message via social media, though I will admit I am rather slow to replying on Facebook. When you receive a reply, know that you are hearing back from ME, not an assistant or a friend or a robot...I can't afford any of those, anyway. (Ha!)

As usual, if you have any questions, comments, or concerns, please do not hesitate to leave a review or reach out to me.

I still read all of my reviews and take your comments in consideration when I'm writing.

I hope you all have a wonderful day, and thank you!

Check me out on Twitter!

https://twitter.com/AuthorKerryHamm

My website:

http://www.authorkerryhamm.com

I'm also on Facebook. Drop a search for Author Kerry Hamm to find my page!

196

Made in the USA
Las Vegas, NV
16 December 2020